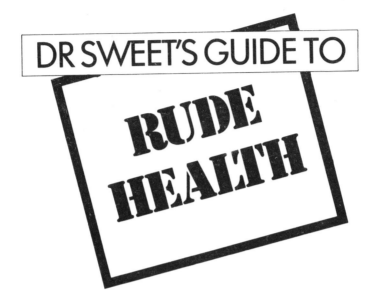

# DR SWEET'S GUIDE TO

## RUDE HEALTH

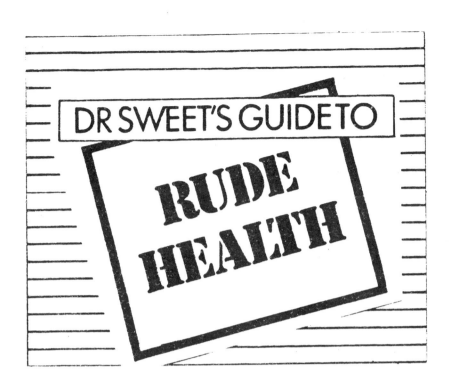

# DR SWEET'S GUIDE TO RUDE HEALTH

Based on the
Channel Four Television series
written by Quentin Brown and Phil Gould

First published in 1987 by Boxtree Limited

Quentin Brown and Phil Gould 1987
Based on the Channel Four series
produced by The Elstree Company

ISBN 1 85283 213 4 hardback
     1 85283 219 3 paperback

Typeset by York House Typographic Ltd, London.
Printed and bound in Great Britain by
Richard Clay Ltd., London
for Boxtree Limited
36 Tavistock Street
London
WC2E 7PB

# Contents

## Minor Ailments

## It's all in the mind: Psychiatry

# Am I Normal, Odd or Bonkers?

## The Ages of Man

## Leisure and Work

## Sexual Medicine

## PS

# List of illustrations

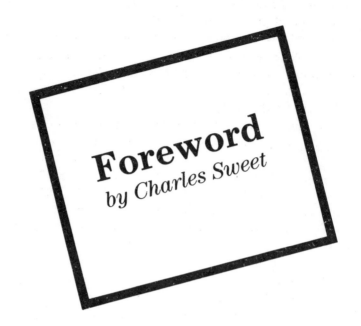

# Foreword
## by Charles Sweet

When I was asked to write this modest tome, I was naturally very pleased and, if I am honest, a little alarmed. For who am I but a humble general practitioner ploughing a lonely furrow amongst the haemorrhoids and herpes of my loyal and devoted patients, hidden away, jealously guarding my privacy and shunning the glare of publicity in a village just off the A369, through a row of cottages, over the level crossing and turn right into the High Street, opposite the 'Jolly Cock'.

I fully realise that the publication of this book might well change my life, perhaps irrevocably. It has never been a wish of mine to become a celebrity, like those ghastly smooth-arsed doctors you see on television. But I fear that the inevitable success of this publication will bring an end to the idyllic peace of a simple and shy man leading a quiet and contented existence, where it is reward enough merely to be worshipped by one's patients.

But I am ready to face the challenge – even if it means opening the odd supermarket or appearing on the Terry Wogan Show, ideally to coincide with publication.

What then, is the purpose of this book? It is directed, I feel, towards the more discerning and intelligent patient – certainly not the belly-aching band of scrimshankers and layabouts who clog up my waiting-room every Monday morning. No, it's for *you* – the high-ranking member of the Diplomatic Corps, just returned from an important mission to the South Pacific, only to find that a rather important and recently used part of your anatomy now bears a painful reminder that unless treated, will remain, rather like a stick of rock, with 'Forever Fiji' emblazoned through it.

This is meant to be a happy book. I think I can guarantee that, apart from a short chapter on 'Sex and the Eighty Year-Old', you are unlikely to die from any of the conditions mentioned in the text.

For was it not Harold Nicholson, the noted essayist and former manager of Tottenham Hotspur, who said: 'It is one of the minor pleasures in life to be slightly ill'?

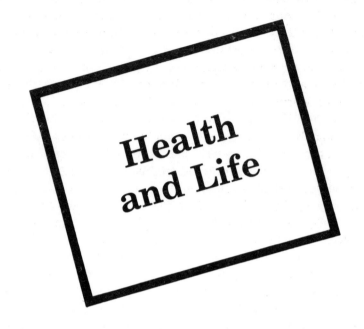

Health
and Life

When we are healthy, our bodies behave like perfectly ordered machines. Powered by 3-litre engines, we purr along in the outside lane, sounding our horns at the foe, flashing our lights flamboyantly to the music of social intercourse. Beneath the gleaming bodywork and the comfortable upholstery we are barely aware of the slip and slide of the complex moving parts that keep us going; valves open and shut, fluid is pumped, filtered, squirted and steamed off, warm rich oils bathe hurtling pistons and miles and miles of slithery bits. And all more or less without our knowledge.

Unfortunately there are machines and there are other machines. The brain, for example, may resemble a sophisticated computer, fully equipped with massive memory banks, or it may be more like a liquidiser, or perhaps even a light bulb.

Physically we differ. Not all of us can be a Mazerati, weaving and dodging life's obstacles in effortless overdrive. Some must content themselves with a humbler passage, edging along the hard shoulder in a Transit van. But there we all are, out on life's thoroughfare, fully taxed and insured, setting off with a full tank of fuel. And I like to think, in quiet moments, that even in the most lumbering, dirty old haulage truck, bound only, perhaps, for the quarry, or to some fish-head depot, God in His Heaven may nonetheless have planted a heart which ticks with the quiet unfailing intricacy of a Swiss clock, sweetly chiming the hours and dreaming of one day meeting a mate – a tractor perhaps, or a small buxom threshing machine.

## Looking After Ourselves

In health, we glow and gleam, our skins are nourished by sun and natural oils, we are rosy, content and regular in our functions. Our hair shines, our teeth are like ivory chisels, our tongues moist and pink. How can we keep them this way?

1 *Emigrating.* Contrary to popular opinion, the Romans first visited our island not to conquer but to gather sphagnum moss for their hanging geranium baskets. Whilst they were rootling round in the bog plants, they were astonished to see pallid, spectral figures issuing out of the mists, clutching kleenexes and blue with chilblains. Terrified, they legged it back to the Adriatic for 'flu jabs' and only later established Ancient Britain as a punishment centre.

Most conquering races have avoided Britain ever since; William the Conqueror only came here as a dare.

There are few obvious examples of the health benefits of

incessant drizzle, hailstorms and impenetrable fog. One is that you tend to lose enthusiasm for cannibalism. This has died out except in parts of Shropshire when it's sunny.

**2** *Self-health.* Much of this book will be devoted to ways of looking after yourself without disturbing the overworked doctor. Essential to this is a grasp of your own biology. Now you may think that understanding the workings of the body is going to involve a lot of work. Well, you're dead right. The whole thing is damned tricky, especially the brain. All you need to know is that your body contains items of extraordinary complexity, such as innards and gizzards, which *you* don't understand but your doctor does.

**3** *Doctors.* All machines need a bit of a going over once in a while. Fuses blow, bits fall off, things won't start or else they won't stop. If this happens to your lawnmower you examine it, tinker about with it and then kick it. Doctors use similar principles. They specialise in the most complex bit of machinery of all. Hubcaps, disbributor heads, whirly bits – your doctor is familiar with every last screw. Don't be afraid of your doctor. Next time your lawnmower breaks down, take it along to him.

## Now We Are Sick

Our climate is not exactly tailor-made for ideal health in the primitive sense; swinging through the tree canopy with bronzed limbs, nibbling nuts and berries and romping with chums in wooded glades is only possible on close, balmy days with close, balmy chums. Long ago the Saxons learned to make the best of things by huddling together in stone dwellings, sniffing up Friar's Balsam and peering out at the rain. These cheerful, enterprising types were, of course, our ancestors, and many of their customs and knowledge have been handed down to us. Few nations better understand the different types of drizzle and can talk for so long about it, and nowhere is there such a detailed popular knowledge of phlegm, catarrh or post-nasal drip. Much of this was woven into sagas until handkerchiefs were eventually introduced by the Plantagenets.

As a people, our expectations of health are traditionally limited. Thus, dreariness of spirit, condensation in major joints and collections of mucus, rattling round any hollow organ communicating with the nose, however remotely, have long been associated with a sense of well-being. At some point, however, people ceased to be naturally phlegmatic in their disposition. One explanation offered by historians is the arrival of money, closely followed by the

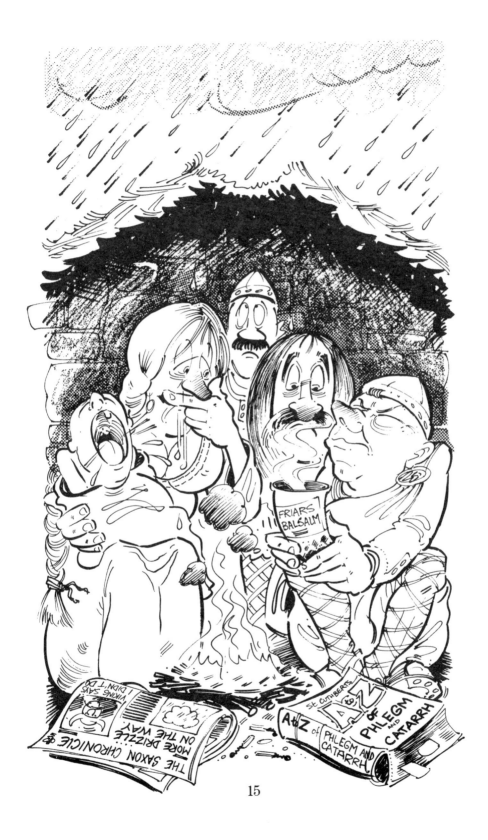

arrival of doctors. Expectations somehow rose; having handed over the entire proceeds of the swede harvest to the doctor and his apothecary, people soon began belly-aching for results. At first it was just foot-powders, ear-syringing and the odd poultice, but in no time at all quite ordinary people were expecting to live beyond twenty-two. The common folk lost their traditional sense of humour. Villages that a century before would have been able to see the funny side of the Black Death began to ruminate intensely about anthrax and threadworms.

Doctors responded to this challenge by developing tools to fight back illness – drawbridges, moats, boiling oil usually discouraged sick people from bringing their germs too close and later the bull mastiff was invented. When the pestilence had finally burnt itself out, it left a more subdued populace who were somewhat ambivalent towards doctors and rats. People were generally more inclined to ask to see a specialist. Doctors sought to regain their intellectual standing in the community by learned pursuits such as robbing graves and dissecting dead bodies. Patients left in their droves.

For doctors this was a time of crisis. Having convinced an entire culture that lice, scabies, boils and running sores were not part of nature's plan but *diseases*, people preferred to tout these ailments to toothless old hags sitting in hovels, dispensing comfrey leaves and frog spittle. In order to regain their monopoly over disease, doctors took on all manner of revolting and unspeakable jobs that nobody else could countenance: draining swellings, lancing boils, probing about in gentlemen's underwear. Resistance caved in; herbalists, palmists, aroma-therapists slunk off into the backwaters whence they have only recently tramped out again.

Doctors had achieved a revolution in public consciousness. It had taken fifteen centuries to civilise the Anglo Saxon peasant into worrying about pre-menstrual tension. Perhaps in another fifteen centuries we'll find a cure.

## Your Heritage

Feeling ill is clearly part and parcel of our Great British Heritage; and we have a duty to posterity to ensure that it keeps its place in the British way of life. For not by Treaties and Declarations of Intent was the Empire welded, but by traipsing across the trade routes spreading mumps and chicken pox. It will indeed be a sad day when we British can no longer feel a bit better for dwelling gloomily upon our aches and pains.

So remember – you are *entitled* to grumble about how awful you feel. It is your birthright. Don't bottle it up. People will only get irritated if you go around looking in peak condition and grinning cheerfully. Better to have a good whinge and be accepted in society. It doesn't matter what it is – hiatus hernia, chapped lips – it needn't be pleurisy or anything serious – but do *try* to do your bit to help us all feel rotten together. The nation works better for it.

Start tomorrow.

Get up, twist your ankle getting out of bed, bring up last night's Horlicks, fling open the curtains and say:

'God, I've got a headache.'

How better to start the day?

## Minor Illnesses

One or more minor illnesses can usually be induced in the first few minutes of the working day. Statistically you have a fair-to-middling chance of actually waking up with one. Prickling sensations in the back of the throat, watery eyes and gummed-up nostrils usually herald the arrival of the common cold, though admittedly the same symptoms may simply be due to a rather rancid pair of pyjamas. A rash is irrefutable evidence that something is wrong and many surgeries will take your word you've got one just from a careful description over the telephone. Describing Laura Ashley wallpaper over the 'phone can sound convincingly like German Measles or even *Pityriasis rosea* – a harmless condition that lasts up to eight weeks.

A little concentration over breakfast is usually all that is needed to locate the bit of you that isn't working properly today. Perhaps it hurts slightly, sounds peculiar if you press on it or shake it, or maybe it's merely gone a bit blue. If a preliminary reconnoitre doesn't reveal anything untoward turn your attention to the plumbing and winding gear. A careful search will almost invariably come up with something to feel one degree under about. A trapped nerve, a slightly blocked tear duct, a barely audible purring noise in the entrails – none is completely valueless as a symptom. If you can find *absolutely* nothing the matter, not even a whisper of dizziness, not so much as a twinge of nausea, if you can't even *imagine* you've got a headache, then you should see a doctor. You could be seriously depressed.

17

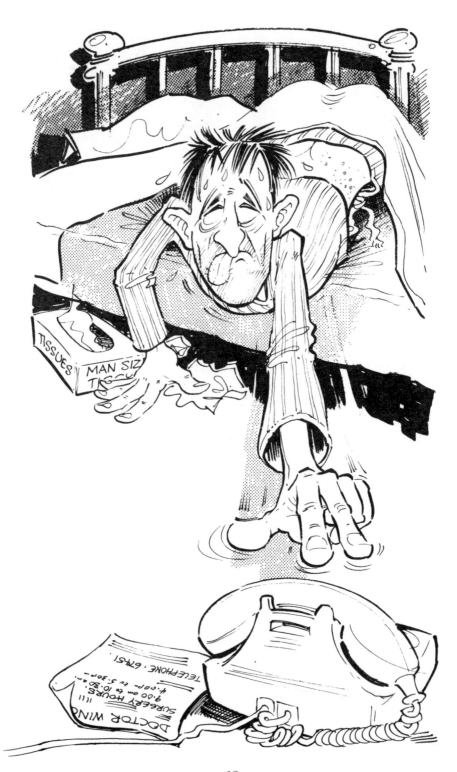

## Why grin and bear it?

Putting up with a minor ailment helps to distinguish us as a race of grumbling stoics. Like the traditional ice-cold bath in the morning, it gives the stiff upper lip something to be stiff about. In times of peril these qualities give the nation its spine and its teeth. Our leaders know this. A nation that has taken itself off to work despite hacking tracheitis for eight months of the year is not going to take kindly to being walloped by the Hun. Moaning about lumbago and fallen arches all helps to maintain our perception of ourselves as 'underdogs', who as we all know, always end up on the winning side.

This is why governments spend billions of pounds a year to pay doctors to diagnose and treat self-limiting illnesses.

## The rules of the game

There must be a minimum level of hypochondriasis for us to function fully in society. Otherwise we'd all bounce around smiling at one another in a thoroughly decadent way. In no time at all we'd be glowing with health and prancing around freezing-cold beaches with no clothes on, just like the Germans do. Nobody would go to work, the National Health would rust and crumble, the economy would fail.

No! This must never happen. A complacently healthy nation is a vulnerable nation. We, on the other hand, thrive on being pale and miserable, dull of wit yet swift in bowel action. Nurture your little aches and pains. And take no notice of those who say there's nothing the matter with you. Just keep coming in your busloads. 9-10 a.m. That's my surgery time – every day, three days a week. Emergencies only on Saturdays and Wednesday evening.

---

### Editor's Note

Dr Sweet is not allowed to advertise, but compassion compels him at least to provide a grid reference for those many people who have written in to join his present happy flock of 5,304 patients. He would not wish to deny his services to any of those anxious to benefit from his years of experience and dedication, especially if they are prepared to go privately. Otherwise, I'm afraid it's a bit of a case of 'dead men's boots' . . .

---

# Getting To See The Doctor

You have woken up with a mortal case of blocked nostril. Your kidneys are making funny noises or you have noticed hair sprouting from the roof of your mouth.

You have consulted a medical encyclopaedia and decided you have Von Girlitz's Syndrome (the first recorded case in a primate for ninety-four years).

Your temperature is 112° Fahrenheit and you were unable to finish your early morning tea because of churning bowel movements.

## A Guide Through the Surgery

### Making an appointment by phone

Assuming you can drag your perspiring body across the floor to a telephone, you will dial the surgery number; it will ring for a few minutes before the phone is picked up. There is then a silence of up to two or three minutes, because the receptionist is very busy and has put down the phone to deal with someone who's being awkward. Eventually, she will pick it up again and say something like, 'Yes, what do you want?'

Don't be discouraged by her tone. This is merely to frighten off non-urgent cases, who will take the hint and apologise for ringing the wrong number. Obviously, receptionists would really like the surgery's number to be ex-directory.

### Surviving the receptionist

Bear in mind that receptionists are often people who have left the SAS because of unsuitability. Or think of them as a cross between a bloodhound and a Doberman. Their job is to sniff out trouble and then deal with it quickly and cleanly.

Let us assume, however, that you have successfully negotiated the first hurdle and the receptionist has not hung up on you. Always sound grateful, or better still, subservient. Don't say anything unnecessarily provocative such as, 'Can I have an appointment, please?' A safer approach might be: 'I know you're extremely busy and it will probably wait, but my little Tommy has climbed into the washing machine and it's now on fast spin. Is there any chance of the doctor coming out or should I call the plumber?'

This stands a very good chance of success and the receptionist would in all probability have the plumber's number.

## Other ways of making an appointment

For those who wish to take the coward's way out in order to avoid actually speaking to the receptionist, the following methods of making an appointment should be considered:

1 Telex.
2 Despatch rider.
3 Brick with message through the window.
4 Appointogram.

## Entering the surgery

Congratulations, you've made it! If you are a newcomer, try to relax. Look around, take in your surroundings. You will see lots of patients sitting about with their heads bowed. But don't be fooled; beneath that seemingly cowed and sullen exterior, there are hearts beating just a little more proudly, because they too have overcome appalling obstacles to be granted an appointment!

Fortified in the knowledge that you are one of the finalists, stride as confidently as you can to the reception area. Knock on the glass partition and announce yourself thus in a clear and steady voice, (receptionists don't react well to weakness): 'I have an appointment with the doctor at 10.30.'

She will then examine the list and, without looking up, say, 'No you haven't!'

Don't be put off by this, as it is a routine ploy just to test you. After letting you sweat for a bit, she will reluctantly admit that, yes, you appear to be right, and instruct you to take a seat. This is the moment you have been waiting for. Only yards away lies your salvation – a welcoming, empty plastic bucket seat. An aeon seems to pass as you stagger towards it. Another three steps and you'll be safe and blissfully anonymous. You reach your haven and smile self-deprecatingly at your neighbour. He looks nervously away. You are about to sink into recumbent peace, when a stentorian blast from the receptionist reminds you that the gap between your derrière and the seat are separated by light years:

'OH YES ... YOU'VE COME TO HAVE YOUR COIL FITTED, HAVEN'T YOU?'

You smile weakly. She has won and you wish you'd never reached puberty.

## The waiting room

If the surgery isn't too busy, you might only have to wait an hour or two to be seen. Even so, you do have to spend it in company with a horrid bunch of people called 'Other Patients'.

This is like sitting down to dinner with a load of uninvited strangers to whom you feel superior. And there's no dinner.

Here are a few guidelines to help you get through this unpleasant experience.

**1** You will notice that, on the whole, nobody will look at one another, except for the occasional sneaky glance. By astute timing, you can get in a few of your own.

**2** Try to guess what's wrong with the other patients. Even better, amuse yourself by imagining that they've all got piles. Have a little rest and then imagine that none of the men are wearing any trousers. By juggling around with these thoughts, you can easily while away the first hour or so of waiting.

**3** Never hold the bit of your body that you've come to see the doctor about.

**4** If you think you're going to die, best do it at home. If done in the waiting-room, it can cause a lot of unnecessary fuss, as well as a good deal of tiresome paper-work for doctor.

**5** Try not to get bolshie just because you've had to spend the morning/afternoon at the surgery. Think of doctor, instead, as the captain of Concorde. He may have been delayed by an air traffic controller's strike in Lisbon or been diverted by bad weather over Alaska. Or he may have overslept.

**6** To pass the hours, treat yourself to another browse through those collector's items from yesteryear, often brought in by doctor at considerable expense. You won't always be lucky but 'The BOAC Year Book' and 'The West Bromwich Hotel Guide' can still occasionally be seen. However, be sure not to ask the receptionist whether she has them in stock. As we have seen, she's very busy and has sharp teeth.

## The moment you've been waiting for

By now you've forgotten why you came. But just as the musings of condemned members of the French aristocracy were interrupted by the cheerful sing-song of a female voice calling out: 'Comte de la Tour. Guillotine number three please,' so your turn, too, will finally come.

This can happen in one of various ways.

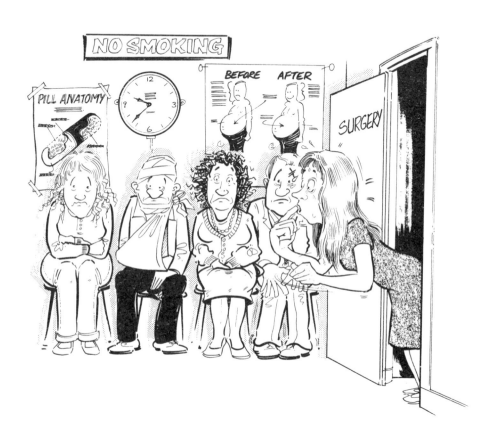

**1** A buzzer will sound. Do nothing. The receptionist will help you on your way with a 'Well go on then!'

**2** A maniacal figure will appear in the doorway, look wildly around and scream 'Next!' Don't be alarmed; it's just doctor running a little late.

**3** A random name will be yelled out. Be alert. When appointments are made, receptionists often take down names in a hurry, so look out for minor variations. If your name is, say, Mr Smithson, your turn could be indicated by the following announcements

*a* Mr Tupolev.

*b* Mrs Koomeraswamy.

*c* Tommy Tucker.

*d* His Grace the Duke of Portland.

**4** A gong sounds. This signifies the start of the surgery's lunch hour. Please show your consideration by being quiet. Doctor will be woken up in time for afternoon surgery.

**5** Everyone else has left and you're still sitting there. This usually means that the surgery's over and you've been forgotten. Best to go quietly home.

## The Doctor

It is terribly important to judge your doctor's mood before you enter.

A few tips. Have there been sounds of shouting coming from his surgery? Has the previous patient come out in tears? When you eventually go in, is *doctor* in tears? Is he swearing/kicking the furniture? Are there droplets of spittle round his lips?

Always remember that doctors are extremely important, clever and busy men. By all means say, 'Good morning, doctor,' or better, 'Good morning, sir.' In lighter moments, they will tell you it doesn't matter how you greet them, but doctors are only human and, if they are honest, they will admit that, apart from putting the relationship on a proper footing, they enjoy receiving deference due to extremely important, clever and busy men.

If you have got the opening greeting correct, he will put you at your ease by looking away, saying 'Hmmph' and indicating the chair all at the same time. This dexterity of mind may well overawe you, but I can tell you it is one of the first things they teach you at medical college.

Never venture a remark such as 'How are you?' This irritates doctors beyond measure. You have broken the protocol. I mean, you wouldn't talk like that to the Queen, would you? There is an order of things, an order that has endured for hundreds of years. I would venture to suggest that if this order had been respected in Russia, that sad country might have saved itself a revolution.

So just keep it to 'Good morning, doctor'.

## Doctor-watching

The doctor's consulting-room can be quite an intimidating place. There's you, the patient, just come off the street, probably anxious and not very intelligent, suddenly confronted by strange sights and smells. Then you sit down in the total silence one always associates with great seats of learning. And there he is.

Now you've probably always thought of doctor as something of a god. And in some ways this is true. Remember, though, that beneath that sometimes stern visage, there is a man who has dedicated his life to the betterment of his fellow human beings, usually in order to get into the masonic lodge.

So you begin to talk. You examine doctor's kindly countenance, searching for some clue as to what is going through that erudite mind. Is it good news? Is it bad news? Is he listening?

Here are some useful tips to help you through those anxious moments.

## What does it mean when . . ?

What does it mean when doctor starts to look serious?
*a* you've got two days to live. *b* He's been looking at the wrong set of notes. *c* He's just broken wind.

What does it mean when doctor starts laughing?
He's having a nervous breakdown. Change your doctor.

What does it mean when doctor starts to break wind?
Your consultation is coming to an end.

What does it mean when your doctor asks you to say, 'Ninety-nine'?
This is an old trick. It has absolutely no meaning but is extremely useful in impressing the patient.

## The sort doctors prefer

Doctors are very busy people. Imagine that he's done an extremely long and tedious morning surgery, before breaking off for a welcome round or two of golf. Imagine that you are the last patient and don't want to make doctor very cross. This is how *not* to do it.

*Patient:*

'Oh . . . I usually see the younger doctor . . . well, the thing is . . . I don't know . . . I seem to be . . . well you know what I mean . . . well of course you do . . . you're a doctor . . . it's just that . . . how can I put it . . . I just don't seem to be able to make any . . . well . . . decisions . . .'

For driving doctor towards homicide, this scores nearly maximum points. Not only is the presentation dull and long winded, but the patient is clearly deranged. Doctors, as a rule, don't like treating loopies.

So, be brief, try to keep your disease simple and preferably above the belt. (See also Clean Underwear.) This is how to do it.

*Patient:*

'Good morning doctor. I've got a very sore throat. I've taken a throat swab and it looks like it's streptococcal. Could I have some Phenoxymethyl penicillin, 250 milligrams, four times a day please?'
*Doctor:*
'Here you are. Goodbye.'

# The Examination

A thorough examination can take anything up to a minute and a half, so help doctor out a bit by avoiding heavy items of corsetry, hose and bodices liable to need a spanner or a monkey-wrench.

When doctor gives you the nod, slip out of your thingummies, go behind the screens and lie nude upon his couch until he is ready to begin the examination. You may have to wait for a while because:
*a* He may be making a telephone call to a private patient.
*b* He has decided to feed his fish.
*c* He may have forgotten you're there.

If someone else comes behind the screens with no clothes on, it means:
*a* Doctor has definitely forgotten you're there.
*b* Doctor has taken leave of his senses.

The examination is traditionally in four parts:

## 1 Inspection
Self-explanatory. It's a bit like choosing wallpaper. Don't be offended if doctor looks disgusted. You probably clash with the carpet.

Doctor will wish to inspect your tongue. Try to avoid this being coated with garlic sausage or other detritus – walking through an automatic car-wash with your mouth open will usually deal with these.

## 2 Percussion
Very important. This is when doctor examines your bongos.

## 3 Palpation
Includes feeling, prodding and rummaging about. A good doctor will palpate you all over. Impostors usually reveal themselves at this stage.

## 4 Auscultation
Just 'listening'. Doctor will get out a big black rubbery thing and lay it under your left breast. Don't be alarmed. This is his stethoscope and he is listening to your heart.

# A word about impostors
Here are a few tips to avoid being examined by unqualified personnel.

## 1 Percussion
A bit like banging on an oil tank to see if it's full or empty. Doctor often percusses your chest or abdomen but it is rare for him to go round the room tapping on radiators and hot-water pipes. Probably prudent to put your clothes back on if he starts doing this.

## 2 Some things doctor rarely carries
   *i* Spirit levels.
  *ii* Blow lamps.
 *iii* Paint stripper.
  *iv* Roofing belt.

## 3 Suspicious bedside manner
*Impostor:* Say 'ninety-nine'.
*You:* 'Ninety-nine'.
*Impostor:* Give a cough.
*You:* Uhuff.
*Impostor:* Um . . .
*You:* Yes?
*Impostor:* Where did you say it hurt?

*You:* Here.
*Impostor:* Oh. Don't suppose I could interest you in a bit of double glazing?
*You:* Pardon?
*Impostor:* Budge up a bit.

## Expressions Often Used by Doctor

| *Expression* | *Meaning* |
| --- | --- |
| I think we might let a specialist have a look at you. | I haven't a clue what's wrong with you. |
| It's probably a virus. | I haven't a clue what's wrong with you. |
| Yes, there's a lot of it about at the moment. | I haven't a clue what's wrong with you. |
| I think we'll try you on some new tablets. | I haven't a clue what's wrong with you. |
| You know, these things tend to clear themselves up. | I haven't a clue what's wrong with you. |
| Ah well . . . you've had a good innings . . . | Ah well . . . you've had a good innings . . . |

## The Urine Sample

At some point in the consultation doctor will probably ask you to pass water for him. You should regard this as a privilege and go prepared. Six cups of tea before you set off for your appointment is suitable for this.

If you are lucky, you will be seen straight away, but it is quite likely that you will have to wait a while, say for three hours. During this time you may notice a mild strangling sensation spreading upwards from the pelvis. Experienced patients recognise these spasms as the firt step in a spiritual journey which we call 'transcendence', or 'rising above'. Transcendence occurs when the bladder rises above the navel; in its full blissful state it is accompanied by a dry mouth, a fullness in the throat and shooting pains in the upper limbs. Novices often rock gently and moan quietly to themselves, but the true stoic achieves transcendence in utter stillness, since sudden movements can be perilous. In this transported state it is possible that you will not even hear your name being called by the receptionist or you may forget what you came to see doctor about. You are now in a state of total catatonia which we call 'karma'. Unaware of the outside world, your pains will eventually recede, a great calm will descend upon you and nurse will come with a mop.

Assuming there are no prior catastrophes and doctor orders you to produce a sample, obey with contrition and humility but do not be flippant. Do not whistle, blow off or make a lot of steam. Above all, stop when the brim of the container has been reached.

If in difficulty, here are some tips. First of all relax, feet apart, breathing gently from the diaphragm. Tilting back from the pelvis, adopt a cherubic pose in the manner of the familiar statuettes that decorate Regency fountains. Try to remember a few snatches of Grieg which conjure three hundred-foot waterfalls plunging into fathomless fiords, or better still, imagine you are a garden sprinkler. If this fails, your doctor will probably co-operate with you by turning on taps and joining you in humming Handel's 'Water Music' and maybe even a few traditional whaling songs. If this doesn't work, doctor will probably be very angry and may sling you off his list.

If you have doubts about your ability to perform, take a sample with you. Though this diminishes somewhat from the occasion, it is less likely to put your doctor in a bad mood than no sample at all. Use a clean jar; fragments of raspberry jam or peanut butter are not normal constituents of urine and may lead to your being put on a kidney machine. On no account take a sample in a bottle marked Liebfraumilch.

## My Kind of Doctor

There are many kinds of doctor to choose from. Ideally, select one who's been to a medical school. Here are a few examples of the types on offer:

### 1 The Old-Fashioned Family Doctor
More of a family friend, really. The old-fashioned 'panel' doctor recalled with fond nausea.

*Advantages*
  *i* Very kind, with big soft white hands.
  *ii* Doesn't shout or raise his voice.
*iii* Rides a nice horse called Dobbin and visits you when you are
      in bed with measles or a cold.
  *iv* Listens to your dolly with his stethoscope.
*Disadvantages*
  *i* Now very old.
  *ii* Believed to be in prison somewhere.

## 2 The Crusty Old Grump

Runs a single-handed practice and likes to do things his own way.
Has no staff but possesses his own microscope.
*Advantages*
  *i* You always see the same person.
  *ii* No receptionist to beat you up.
*Disadvantages*
  *i* Only ever sees hairs down his microscope.
  *ii* Believes everybody has syphilis.

## 3 The Highland Flinger

Charges round the glens in a Morris 18 with lengths of enema
tubing flapping in the wind. Does absolutely everything himself.
Lives in a huge mansion with a housekeeper. Sleeps in an iron
lung. Takes out appendixes on the kitchen table and delivers all
his patients' babies. In extremis will personally row you across the
Sound to the Cottage Hospital.
*Advantages*
  *i* The complete doctor. Fears no emergency.
  *ii* Always jolly.
*Disadvantages*
  *i* Doesn't believe in painkillers but will let you bite on a radish.
  *ii* Giving birth in the bottom of a boat in a Force 9.
*iii* Frequently pissed.

## 4 The Good Listener

Earnest, caring, understanding. *Your* time is *his* time. Doesn't just
fob you off with a prescription. You feel you can really talk to him.
*Advantages*
  *i* Been on some sort of course to do with sex.
  *ii* Will listen to you rabbiting on all day.
*Disadvantages*
  *i* Probably on drugs.

## 5 The Workers' Cooperative Anarchist Health Clinic

Not exactly *a* doctor but more of a healing group. You explain your most intimate personal difficulties to several people at a time, one of whom may be a doctor.

*Advantages*

i A very good consciousness – raising group on constipation on alternative Mondays.

*ii* No great sense of equality.

*iii* No men or pigs admitted.

*iv* Only alternative healing techniques used, e.g. organically grown potatoes.

*Disadvantages*

i Not covered by BUPA.


# 'Have I Got . . .'

## Some Easy Diagnostic Tests

### 1 . . . Worms?

An unpleasant condition often picked up while bending down to do weeding. A good diagnostic test is to take an early morning stroll. If you find you are followed around by blackbirds and robins, the signs are not good. Consult your vet.

### 2 . . . Long to Live?

A good clue is whether your next of kin are showing more than a usual interest in your condition.

Try not to trouble your doctor with this one. Best to look up a medical dictionary.

### 3 . . . Scurvy?

Often caused by hospital food. Consult a dental expert. With his specialist knowledge, he'll be able to tell you whether your teeth have been dropping out.

### 4 . . . Bubonic Plague?

The signs here can be hard to elucidate. Have you been feeling a little below par? Do your friends never seem to turn up when you throw a dinner party? Does that tube always seem to empty the moment you sit down? People can be very hurtful when it comes to the Plague. See also Black Death.

### 5 . . . An Appointment?

This is often asked by the receptionist when you phone up thinking you may be suffering a heart attack.

### 6 . . . A Normal Sex Life?

A recent study has shown that the average couple make love eleven or twelve times a night, with the male often taking two or three partners at a time.

Whether you measure up to this is for you to decide, but bear in mind that it was based on an ordinary family of West African baboons.

### 7 . . . Delusions of Grandeur?

There is nothing wrong with setting your sights high. Where would Genghis Khan have got if he'd decided to be a dentist? The important thing is to make your targets realistic ones. For instance, if you are only averagely intelligent, there would be little point in trying to become, say, a doctor. Why not try dentistry?

### 8 . . . Hereditary Telangectiasis?

I don't know.

### 9 . . . Clean Underwear?

If you're going to see doctor, do take a peek.

### 10 . . . To Go To Work?

Getting a sick note from doctor depends on your condition and his politics. For myself, I can only say that this country has lost its greatness because we've become a nation of shirkers. So I have to tell you that I am no easy touch when it comes to lead swingers who come whining to me for their little piece of paper.

That is not to say I'm stony-hearted about these things. Here are a few conditions which would at least stand a fair chance of success:

1 Heart/lung transplant.

2 Injuries pursuant to non-opening of parachute.

3 Private patients.

### 11 . . . My Prescription Money?

Well, have you?

### 12 . . . An Undersized Gland?

This is probably the most common fear held by the adult male. Over and over they come to us – men who are often too embarrassed to put their innermost fears into words. Under expert guidance, however, the truth will usually out.

'Doctor, you see . . . I'm worried about the size of my thyroid.' Mere confiding often helps, for this is usually a deep-seated and long-held neurosis. Thyroid counselling can be beneficial, and the wife is vital in repairing shattered self-esteem. So can I, therefore, reassure all my male readers that intensive studies have shown that your married life is totally unaffected by the size of your thyroid?

32

Having said that, I know what I'd prefer if I had to choose between a squidgy little one and a real whopper.

## Should I Give Doctor a Present?

Being a doctor is a vocational profession, so called because it often starts off as a holiday job.

'Do I give my doctor a present?' Let me assure you that the last reason doctors become doctors is so that they can be rewarded by material things. No, their motives are rather loftier (e.g. Helping Mankind).

However, doctors are no different to anyone else and just like old Joe Soap in the High Street, he has everyday responsibilities, like the upkeep of the villa, private education of the kids; membership fee at the golf club, that sort of thing.

So by all means give money, but to avoid embarrassment, can I suggest the following sliding scale for gifts? Bear in mind this is only a rough guide.

| | |
|---|---|
| Syringing out ears. | Jar of honey. |
| Rashes, itches, PMT. | Bottle of port (vintage). |
| Urinary tract infection. | Bottle of Bollinger (preferably '57). |
| Runny nose, diarrhoea, vomiting. | Smoked salmon or quail's eggs. |
| Athlete's foot. Anything involving pus. | Pâté. |
| Curing of multiple personality. | Shares in British Telecom (1,000 shares per personality). |
| Bringing back from the dead. | A small mention in the Will (if subsequently applicable). |

## Nurse

Few pronouncements are likely to strike greater dread into the God-fearing heart than the terrible words which signal your transportation to the 'treatment room'.

A silence has fallen upon the consultation. Doctor is pursing his lips; they have gone strangely thin. The clock ticks threateningly. Your mind races.

At last, after what seems an eternity, your sentence is pronounced. Quietly, ominously, almost with sadness:

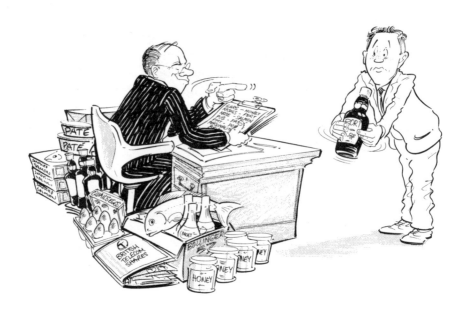

'I think you'd better go and see –'

'Aaaaaargh!!!' Your tongue has sprung suddenly into terrible, shrill life.

'– nurse . . . .'

A haze falls over you, like a curtain coming down. Voices ring distantly in your ears. You are led away.

She has been here as long as anybody can remember. Once, when a girl, it is said that she worked in a hospital, long since condemned. Her echoing tread through Men's Surgical may even have quickened a few pulses and raised a few temperatures in those far-off days before her reputation with the flatus tube was established in the annals of tyranny.

Perhaps the years of disinfecting treatment trolleys got to her, or the constant cries of 'Nurse . . . Nurse . . . I've finished!' Maybe it was the ill-starred fumble in the laundry room with that cad of a surgical registrar. Something must have happened to change this slip of a girl, the blushing forget-me-not of the sluice, into the scourge that would have reduced even cabinet ministers to falsifying their bowel charts.

And now she is here. Lurking in her terrible twilight zone midway between science and medieval torture. Fevered hands propel you in. The door slams behind you. You are alone. In her domain.

Your eyes scan the great brown bottles – Eusol, Ipecac, Carbolic, Antihelminth mixture. And *there*! The notorious *ladles*! Sickened, you avert your gaze. But magnets seem to draw it now to a trolley, set with various lengths of orange, rubber tubing and bits of paraffin gauze. You wonder what the nozzles are for . . . She couldn't *possibly*! . . . Could she?

Panic grips you again. You try to remember what you said in your will. Whether you were nice to the wife and kids when you left them. Tears well up as you peer into the glass cabinet with its probes. In an instant you decide on flight. Out! Out to the fresh cool air, to the birdsong, to the trees. Too late! From nowhere she has pounced. A vast polythene apron suddenly fills the landscape, blotting out the light. A throat swab hurtles through space and disappears to the hilt somewhere beyond your shrieking lips. A great hairy arm muffles your moans. Endlessly the swab sweeps back and forth, searching every cranny for signs of bacterial life, prodding, scraping, gouging.

A moment! The light floods in! Sanctuary! You can breathe again. But the incipient scream for mercy is strangled as it leaves your lips.

'Nnnnnngyaaah!' A second swab, swift as an Exocet, has sped past your defenceless nostrils and up to the soft underbelly of the brain.

Tears scorch your eyelids, streaming on to the floor. You think fondly of the orange, rubber tubes. From within your clammy palm you prise out the crumpled note doctor has given you, proffering it weakly with your last vestiges of strength and courage.

With puzzled, worried eyes, she picks her way across the letters.

'There's been a mistake!' The words croak from your shattered frame.

A pause. She looks sorry. Something resembling a smile brushes across her thick, rude lips.

'Come for a blood test?' she growls.

She reaches for a syringe the size of a strip lamp. You swoon the swoon of the dead.

## NHS or Private?

This is a difficult area for me to talk about. As you know, I run a busy practice that is overwhelmingly NHS, and am more than happy to do so. That is not to say that I don't have just a sprinkling of private patients who force their attentions on me from time to time. I have tried to ward them off, but you know, one does tend to become a prisoner of one's reputation. I only console myself with the fact that there would be far more of these accursed people if I didn't have the good fortune to practise in what is, thankfully, still a fairly grubby area.

Because you see, it makes not a jot of difference to me who comes into my surgery – whether it's Sir Nigel Toft, who lives high on the hill and who, not as often as I'd like, graces me with his presence and sadly has a recurring and very lucrative disease – or old Joe Soap, who lives in a hovel by the railway sidings and comes to see me every Monday, whining about his war service, as well as leaving dirty great muddy footprints all over my extremely expensive carpet.

No, I take people as I find them.

I would be a liar and a hypocrite, however, if I didn't say that private treatment is not without *some* worth. And if there are any of you out there, who, for moral or religious reasons, absolutely insist on private treatment, I feel it would be a dereliction of duty if I were to shun your needs and 'equally invidious of me to withhold what it is in my power to give. A quick phone-call will do it – just mention you've got the ackers and I'll usually be with you in less than half an hour.

To reassure my many and loyal patients that I am totally open-minded about the whole business, let us weigh the comparative advantages.

## Twenty advantages of private treatment

**1** You may call doctor by his first name.

**2** You can insist that he warms his hands before intimate examination.

**3** You are totally justified in buying a doctor a considerable 'thank you' present.

**4** You can choose your own operation from a brochure.

**5** You can insist on an anaesthetic.

**6** You can often get a free holiday for three major operations or six minor ones.

**7** You can insist that your surgeon comes from a good family.

**8** You can insist that your surgeon has done your op. at least once before.

**9** You can be rude to anyone and they still have to smile because you're paying.

**10** You can pay cash and get a 10% discount.

**11** You can insist that nurse wears black stockings and suspenders.

**12** If you're paying enough, you can insist that your surgeon wears black stockings and suspenders.

**13** You can insist on doctor always telling you you're going to pull through.

**14** If you do snuff it, you are entitled to sue for loss of earnings and inconvenience.

**15** Private clinics nearly always sterilise their instruments.

**16** You may insist on inspecting the surgeon's fingernails.

**17** In an emergency, such as cardiac arrest, the clinic will often send round a chauffeur-driven Mercedes. Electric windows and central locking come as an optional extra.

**18** Green Shield stamps.

**19** You are allowed to keep your own pyjamas.

**20** You nearly always get your clothes and belongings back afterwards.

**21** You can insist on your surgeon not smoking.

# Twenty advantages of the NHS

1
2
3
4
5
**6** Everyone gets treated equally, I suppose.
7
8
9
10
11
12
13
14
15
16
17
18
19
20

*__Editor's Note.__ Dr Sweet doesn't appear to have completed this section. Repeated phone-calls and letters have met with no response.

# About Myself

My publisher has asked me if I might say a few words about myself. My first instinct, of course, was to demur, for this book is about *you*, and all the nasty things that can go wrong with your body.

But on reflection, I realised that there may well be many of you out there – high achievers from decent families – who might wish to join the hallowed masonry of the medical profession, and it would be churlish of me, would it not, if I did not at least tell you a little of myself, if only to show that a man from humble origins can overcome seemingly insurmountable obstacles to become a respected and much-loved member of the community.

My parents originally came from the North-East, but in common with many others of the middle-classes, were driven from the land of their forebears because they couldn't stand the accent any longer. A case of too much 'Fishee in the Dishee' making them wishee for a nichee somewhere else.

My great uncle Crabtree had already installed himself in northern Hertfordshire. He had done very well for himself in the building trade and asked my parents to join him. Now my parents were naive and simple folk, and not surprisingly were somewhat dazzled by the bright lights and bustle of a place like Tring. Least of all did they realise that having sunk all their funds into Uncle Crabtree's business empire, great troubles lay ahead.

You see, Crabtree, although basically an honest man, was somewhat vague about the finer points of the building trade, such as foundations, so that one by one, or more accurately, street by street, his revolutionary 'Luxury Pre-Fabs' tended to last for a few months before sort of falling down. This was not good for business, and natives of the area still talk in hushed tones of the 'Great Crash of '48'.

Crabtree dealt with the crisis by emigrating to Brazil. Mother and father were left penniless, but fate now took a hand when we were taken in by Old Doctor Pettigrew, a kindly man with a penchant for the drugs cupboard.

'Snorter' Pettigrew, as he was known, treated us all as his own, employing mother and father as cook and butler.

It was through this great healer that I spent some of my happiest days and felt the first stirrings of a medical calling. I would lie on my bed for hours, flipping through some of the special magazines he lent me, stopping every so often to listen to old Snorter screaming at his patients with exhortations to fight the good fight and exalt in the Lord, as he force-fed them on castor oil and syrup of figs, which he found so efficacious in the treatment of anything from gout to gallstones.

'Never forget, my boy,' he'd tell me, 'give them what they least want and they won't be back for a while.' These words have been an inspiration to me to this very day.

It was at such a moment that I knew I wanted to be a doctor.

Time went by . . . long, glorious summers spent idyllically by the river, poring over any medical literature I could find. Storing knowledge that one day I knew I would need. Come 1955 and I was London bound to medical school.

My first days at St Olaf's were, I freely confess, deeply shocking to me. The sight of my fellow students – some with long hair and all, I may add, from far less humble backgrounds than I – cavorting around the hallowed portals of that great seat of learning, filled me with the greatest disgust and abhorrence. Lewd songs, with unmentionable words, sung in the company of equally disgusting females among great puddles of beer, were not what I had come to expect. I was there to learn and by God I did.

This did not, I need add, endear me to my so-called colleagues. 'Toady Sweet' was my given name and they never let me forget it as they rattled my windows late at night, while I struggled in my room with the mysteries of the autonomic nervous system and the delights of tendons and ligaments.

But I had an armour stronger than any rattly old window. You see, I was going to be a surgeon and no one was going to stop me.

I suppose, like all dreams, mine was just a fervent desire, waiting to be dashed to pieces on the rocks of fate.

Of course, I realise I wasn't and am not the easiest of men. Don't suffer fools and all that stuff, and my downfall, no doubt, was that I didn't choose to be 'one of the boys'. Singing rugby songs and throwing up every Friday night was not, if you will pardon the metaphor, my cup of tea.

Of course, they're all surgeons now, easily esconced in their little rooms in Harley Street, complete with wall to wall Arabs, all glued to the crapper worrying about oil prices.

Dear oh dear, I seem to have got rather emotional, don't I? Well, I wouldn't want you to think I've become bitter about it all, because I haven't. No, not me. I'm quite happy where I am, thank you very much. Quite happy. Because I'm dealing with the *real* world, *real* people in my little neck of the woods. And I don't mind admitting that I'm proud of the little business I've built up.

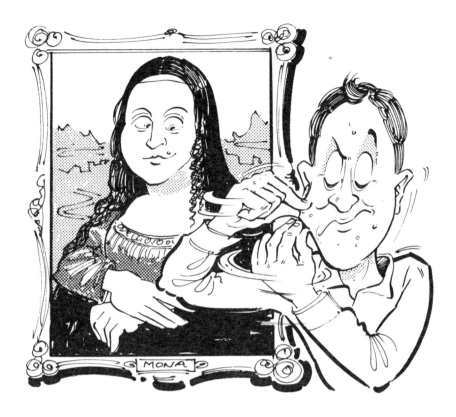

MONA

You see, a busy general practice is like a local garage. Patients coming in through my door aren't looking for a full service – they want a full tank, top-up of oil and water, tyres checked and off they go. If they want a spot of in-car valeting and their ash-trays hoovered out, they can push off to Harley Street. My patients don't come here for a chat and quite frankly, nor do I. In out, in out, shake it all about – pat them on the backside and the next customer please. To put it in a nutshell, I'm at my surgery to cure boils and bunions, not to raise Lazarus.

So, dear reader, next time you go to see your doctor, remember that despite his austere demeanour and awe-inspiring presence, you might be dealing with a child of circumstance, who grew up in a world of might-have-beens . . . a garden seeded with forget-me-nots that somehow came up as nettles. So be gentle with him.

Or he's liable to start shouting at you . . .

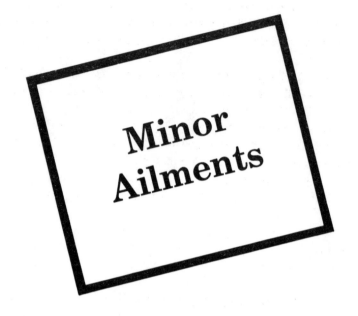

# Minor Ailments

# Spots

Spots, let's face it, can be a problem and indeed can ruin one's credibility. What would the Mona Lisa have looked like if that enigmatic smile had been accompanied by a red and purple whopper associated with an infected hair root nestling just above her top lip?

Although this particular curse can be associated with dietary imbalance, allergy or hormonal changes, the most common cause, I'm afraid, is that you just happen to be a spotty person.

It may be you can live with this, but when you begin to realise that your friends are bringing around parties of total strangers just to have a look, it really is time it went.

This can be a quite exciting moment, for it represents an opportunity to indulge in a bit of your very own surgery. Here's what you do!

Get up nice and early and put on some old clothes. Go into the largest room in the house and cover all the furniture with ground sheets. Criss-cross the windows with strong masking-tape and you are ready!

Shut your eyes tightly, grip the beast firmly and give it a sharp tweak in a clockwise or anti-clockwise direction, depending on its thread. Put on some loud music, for you may need to yell, scream and dance about a bit. After your brain has cleared, you will experience a calmness only experienced by Tibetan monks. Finally, make yourself a sandwich and take a week off work.

# Jock Rash

This unpleasant condition was not, as some have thought, brought to this country by Celtic Hordes, or indeed, Celtic Fans. It was first detected following a goodwill visit of a team of Bulgarian women shot-putters.

Say what you like, these magnificent girls, brought up on a strict diet of new potatoes and anabolic steroids, were a fine sight as they hurled the massive sphere out of Wembley Stadium – breaking world records and shattering windows in nearby Harlesdon.

Sadly, many of them began to show the dangers of using muscle-building drugs by subsequently sprouting anesteric bolloids. Some defected and settled down here, repaying their debt to their adopted country by building the M28, where their work as earth diggers is still remembered.

What is it? Well, just as pink little babies get similar problems, usually from undetected accidents in the nappy department, so too do adult sportsmen, especially second row forwards and often for the same reason.

So if you're, say, an English forward, playing at Cardiff Arms Park and you feel the excitement of the occasion is getting the better of you, a quiet word with the ref is usually all that's required for him to call a temporary halt while you waddle off in the direction of the trainer's trench. Indeed, the 50,000 Welsh crowd will often help you on your way with a hearty cheer, followed by three verses of 'Men of Harlech', while you do the necessary and change into something more comfortable.

## Amnesia

Amnesia can be a very difficult condition to treat, not least because by the time sufferers present themselves at the surgery, they have usually forgotten what they have come for. This can be very annoying to the busy general practitioner. I generally stick them in the waiting room in the hope that it will ring a bell and help them remember they've got amnesia. This can have complications, since the moment they remember they've got amnesia, they forget what their name is. Whilst pondering on this conundrum, they then forget they've got amnesia again and wonder what they're doing there. They finally wander into your consulting room and sit there waiting for you to discover what's wrong with them and what their name is. This can go on for some hours.

I generally break this impasse by selecting a name and a disease for them. Fortified with the knowledge that doctor has cured them of whatever it is they're meant to have had, they leave the surgery, light-footed and with not the faintest clue where they live. They tend to look for somewhere familiar, often ending up in the British Museum, trying to persuade the Director kindly to leave his house.

Amnesiacs have played absolute havoc with history down the ages. Sir Alexander Fleming, for example, had worked for years on trying to discover the aspirin. Infuriatingly, just as success beckoned, he forgot what he was doing and discovered penicillin by mistake. He compounded the problem by going to Sweden and turning up at the wrong ceremony, baffling the scientific world by carrying off the Nobel Prize for Poetry.

# Body Odour

A lot of uninformed and misguided information has tended to obscure the fact that body odour actually has a function. You see, BO is part of our Body Language. It is an absolute tragedy that we spend countless millions of pounds each year merely in an attempt to hide or disguise what our body is trying to tell other people. Let me explain. In the Old Days, before you and I were born, primitive men went around squirting what was admittedly a fairly pungent liquid on trees, plants, or their furniture. What they were doing was *marking their territory*. The result? There were no wars, let alone arguments as to where your territory started or ended – because any attempt by an intruder to encroach upon your patch was rudely brought to an end as he ran off vomiting.

Alas, these extremely useful scent glands evolved themselves into a cul-de-sac and disappeared. Now, I'm not suggesting that modern man, even if he had them, should still use them – it would be ludicrous, for example, for suburban man to rush out and spray his privet hedge every time a stranger passed, especially in a place like Haywards Heath.

All I am saying is that BO is part of our heritage. So next time you find yourself sitting near to a rather sweaty specimen on the tube, take solace in the knowledge that you are sitting next to a living fossil. Do not, however, share this information with him as he could well punch you.

# Unwanted Hair

This can be a real menace, especially for women. Imagine how the socialite feels after she's spent a fortune on a sensational new dress, set off with a dazzling string of pearls from Cartier's, only to have the whole effect ruined by a five o'clock shadow.

The only helpful advice I can give for these unfortunate people is to try to accept it as part of yourself. You can't hide it – so use it.

Here are a few fashionable suggestions:

If you're slender and rather willowy, a devastatingly effective addition is provided by the zapata moustache – streaked, if necessary. On the other hand, if you're a bit on the short and dumpy side, you can be simply transformed by a smart little goatee beard. The effect is said to be quite extraordinary. If you're just a simple country girl, a small Hitler moustache can look quite charming, although one might add that if you're just a simple

45

country girl, it doesn't really matter what you look like.

Joan of Arc, in common with nearly all French women, had terrible problems with facial hair, which seriously eroded her credibility as a national leader and led to her being called 'The Old Maid of Orleans'. This nearly caused the Pope to take back her sainthood. Fortunately, she managed to pull her socks up (another silly attribute for a saint) and, as every schoolboy knows, ended her days in a blaze of glory. What is not generally known is that when they tied her to the stake, she refused the offer of a final cigarette and demanded a decent shave instead, before they lit the twigs.

## Déjà Vu

This common phenomenon is totally unexplained, but should not cause any undue worry. Some psychic authorities maintain that it is a reminder of a previous incarnation; but this is doubted by orthodox medicine. This common phenomenon is totally unexplained, but should not cause any undue worry. Some psychic authorities maintain that it is a reminder of a previous incarnation; but this is doubted by orthodox medicine.

If in doubt, consult your doctor your doctor.

## Breaking Wind

This can be a most distressing condition, especially if it has gained such a hold that you have totally lost control. This can have particularly grave repercussions if you hold high public office, such as Black Rod.

Historically, the Romans have a lot to answer for. Was it not they whose gatherings were dominated by their guests signifying approval of the soirée by letting out a blast before they'd even got on to the grapes?

Look, no one wants to be a kill-joy, but bearing in mind that environmentalists, perhaps over-zealously, are becoming increasingly active against those considered to be in breach of the Clean Air Act, may I suggest that you at least cut down on the following? Globe artichoke soup. Indirectly responsible, according to some, for Dutch Elm disease.
Petit pois. Difficult to translate accurately, but 'Little Poison' is fairly close.
Hurriedly eaten cashew nuts. Said to be the most frequent reason for the dog being unfairly kicked.

Bubble & Squeak.   No explanation needed, I fear.

Is there anything that is totally safe? Unfortunately, the answer must be 'no'. True, some foods do have a low wind-factor, but sitting down to a plate of mashed potato, kiwi fruit and fennel would seem to many too high a price to pay.

Indeed, if one wanted confirmation of the miracle of the human body, one need only contemplate the fact that something as beautiful as Escalopes de Veau en Papillote, followed by Les Oeufs à la Neige au Citron and washed down with a bottle of Château Lafite, can manifest itself so catastrophically at the other end.

## Insomnia

It is sometimes a consolation for insomniacs to know that people of a more intellectual nature often need less sleep.

One can imagine Einstein tossing and turning, having just crowned years of research by coming up with $e = mc^2$ and spending the rest of the night trying to remember what 'e' stood for.

On the other hand, if you're not trying to solve any great problem and you still find sleep elusive, the chances are that you are not a genius and probably quite stupid.

What you must do is *relax*. I don't just mean when you get into bed. Start doing it long before you think of retiring.

Have a quiet evening, maybe a glass or two of your favourite wine. Put your feet up on the sofa and listen to some Beethoven or Brahms.

Your eyelids will start to feel very heavy and you will start to feel so, so *comfortable*. Take a small stroll round the garden, savouring the aroma and stillness of the night. Then make that wonderful journey up the stairs. Undress slowly, contemplating the beauty of life, and climb into your warm and soft womb. Your head sinks into the pillow. All is peace. All is peace.

At this point the back of one of your legs, just in the crease behind the knee, starts to itch. Soon it is joined by another. Only this one, generally located about six inches below the back of the neck and therefore just out of reach, feels like there's a rumba being performed by a formation dance team of centipedes.

You are now rapidly falling awake. You change position to gain some relief. But the centipedes have now moved on, only reappearing to perform the pasa doble in an area where no man should ever scratch.

Because your feet are getting hot, you stick them out of the side of the bed so that the configuration of your body, having started off at a restful six o'clock position, has now contorted itself into a quarter to four.

The centipedes are doing a lap of honour inside your left ear. You now tear the sheets off and with the air resonating to screamed obscentities, you thrash about – scratching, swearing, sobbing – until you realise the alarm-clock is ringing and your partner is informing you that it's your turn to make the breakfast.

# Snoring

If anything highlights the imperfection of Man, it is the squeaking, piercing, scratchy, throaty, stentorian baying, snorting and croaking that generically add up to Snoring. By day, you might be Professor of Fine Arts, but come the small hours, you can become aurally undistinguishable from a warthog.

## The Warthog

Generally speaking, the Warthog doesn't muck about with niceties – the moment that head hits the pillow, it starts.

Hggh . . . Hggh . . . Hggh.

Unvarying and unstoppable. A well-aimed dig or kick produces nothing more than a temporary respite, before the dreadful rhythm of rasp continues on its midnight melody. The only relief for the long-suffering partner comes when the awful sound reaches such a crescendo that it wakes the snorer up as well. Hence:

Hggh . . . Hggh . . . Hggh . . . *Hggh – Wassat?* . . . Snggffefer . . . Fnoofer . . . Hggh . . . Hggh . . .

This will continue until the alarm-clock goes off, when our professor will wake from his porcine pillow-talk, refreshed and raring to go.

## The Snorer/Philosopher

The tragedy of snoring is that the silent partner is inevitably a light sleeper. It is also fairly obvious that one snorer will not wake up another. If the Warthog can make life hell for his spouse, so too can the Snorer/Philosopher.

It is 4 a.m. The husband's normal snoring pattern 'Frmmmp . . . Frmmmp . . . Frmmmp . . .' is suddenly interrupted by the deeply significant philosophical enquiry, posed thus: 'Frmmmp-ah . . .

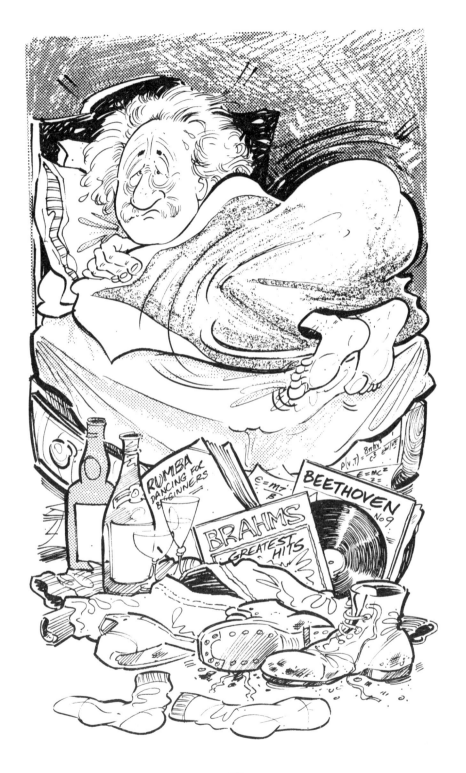

Frmmmmp-ah . . .' This denotes a sense of increasing unease. The snoring is now interspersed with agonised cries of 'Why . . . I mean? . . . It's not! . . . Can't be! . . . Besides, it isn't!!!' The wife jolted awake and thoroughly alarmed, tries questioning him and a mad conversation ensues punctuated by 'Why did you say "It isn't?"' 'What isn't?' 'You said "It isn't".' 'I didn't!' 'You did!' 'You're lying.' 'Oh, shut up!' and similar endearments, batted to and fro into the wee hours, effectively robbing both parties of any further sleep.

So what is the solution? Ear-plugs, a separate room or house? I suppose homicide is the only certain cure. But there's always the chance you'll spend the rest of your days locked up in a cell with a Warthog.

## Baldness

Let's face it, no one much likes going bald, particularly women. Can anything be done about it? Certainly. Here are a few ideas.

### 1. The Naturopathic Transplant

Cut some chunks of hair from your remaining thatch, (or a friend's, preferably with hair of roughly the same colour), separate them into strands and stick them on carefully with a fifty per cent solution of denture adhesive.

*Advantages*
   Cheap and cheerful.

*Disadvantages*
   a) Can look very silly.
   b) Doesn't work.

### 2. Chest Hair Transplant

This is far more scientific than the above method. The hairs are ripped out complete with follicle and sown into the bare patches.

*Advantages*
   Very naturalistic, since it often comes with its own supply of dandruff.
*Disadvantages*
   Can be difficult for women.

## 3. Pubic Hair Transplant

*Advantage*
   Can be a lot of fun.

*Disadvantages*
   a) Difficult to match if you've got straight hair.
   b) Crabs.

## 4. The Three-Strand Trick
Take your three remaining strands of hair, either from the back or side of your head, grease them well and smear them across your pate, stapling them in if necesary. You won't fool anybody, but at least it shows you're not going down without a fight.

*Advantages*
   a) You're not cheating.
   b) You'll give people a good laugh.

*Disadvantage*
   An insensitive barber can ruin years of work. Tell him you only want a bit off.

# Wigs

It is a little-known fact that for years Queen Victoria was almost completely bald. Needless to say, if word of this had got out, within months the Empire would have collapsed.

Very few people were privy to the secret. Gladstone was called in to comment on her appearance, but sycophantically ventured that he thought the Empress Queen was looking as serenely beautiful as ever, and was promptly fired.

It was Disraeli who, drawing on his experience in the schmutter trade, came up with a brainwave. Why not tack a wig to fit inside her crown? It was an immediate success, although an absolute sod to get on.

Nowadays, great strides have been made in the manufacture of wigs, inasmuch as everyone still knows you've got one, but you don't look quite so silly.

Still, there are certain rules that should be adhered to if you wish to avoid embarrassment.

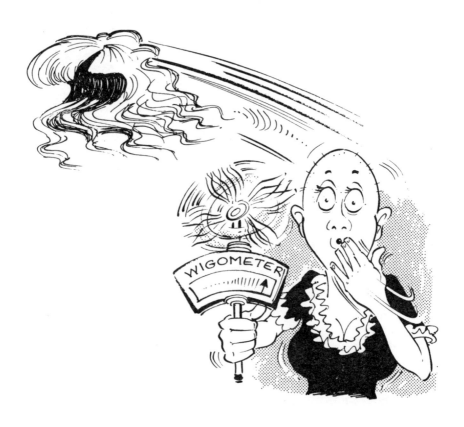

1. Always walk in a straight line, with *no* sudden turns.
2. Before venturing out, check the weather forecast. *Never* go out in windy conditions.
3. Review your sexual techniques. Sudden and violent movements can cause it to fall over your face, bringing coitus to an abrupt end.
4. Always use the stairs. Avoid fast-moving lifts.

A new breakthrough has been claimed by the makers of the revolutionary 'Edith Cavell Five-in-One Hairpiece'. This really is state of the art stuff, consisting as it does of wig, spectacles, false nose, nipples and truss, all held in place by an elaborate system of Velchrome. Unfortunately, it has been reported that sufferers with hay-fever using this contraption have ended up in the Intensive Care Unit.

# Cramp

All of us have suffered from cramp at one time or another. It is caused by an involuntary tightening of a muscle, often the calf, and to the onlooker its onset can be rather startling. One moment you are behaving like a perfectly normal and rational human being and the next you are thrashing about on the floor, screaming with pain and yelling obscenities.

Here are some examples where such an attack would be less than convenient:

**1.** You are the Archbishop of Canterbury about to perform the Coronation.

**2.** You are about to be knighted.

**3.** You are giving a graveside eulogy.

**4.** You are the Prime Minister, reassuring the nation that it hasn't been taken over by aliens.

Normally, your muscles have a soft but firm feel, not unlike a rather succulent kipper. When cramp strikes, however, it undergoes sudden spasm and ends up feeling more like a rollmop herring.

Cramp commonly occurs in a variety of settings:

## 1. Hot Climate

Thought to be due to excessive sweating, although long periods of clenching a camel hump between your knees certainly doesn't help.

## 2. Exhausting Physical Exercise

Depends on the individual. Those with a low threshold can get violent attacks whilst fishing. Treatment is difficult if you're clad in thigh-length gumboots, but then so are a lot of things.

Footballers often get cramp during debilitating nil-nil draws. Two varieties are well-described.

### *i* The 'Wembley Jinx'

The player charges his way from the half-way line on one leg and hurls himself into the back of the net, usually to avoid being substituted.

### *ii* The 'Wembley Hoodoo'

Much worse. Players (usually several at a time) lie prostrated in the penalty area, point one leg at the referee and utter piteous cries of 'urrghooodooh'.

## 3. Deep Slumber

Notorious. Often interrupts spiffing dreams. A sleeping partner or colleague can help by offering you something to bite on. This often brings about relief, divorce, rabies or blood-poisoning, depending on the choice of partner and the bit of anatomy you have sunk your teeth into.

## 4. Coitus

Cramp is often mistaken for climactic sexual ecstasy. Don't encourage this belief as you may be asked to do it again; it is much harder to fake than orgasm and far more painful. As with fishing, avoid thigh-length gumboots.

## 5. Groin Cramp

Peculiar to males. This tends to occur following singularly unsuc-cessful forays with members of the opposite sex. It generally wears off after a fortnight of cold showers and a diet of nuts and raisins.

## 6. Proctalgia Fugax

This literally means 'fleeting pain in the bum' and is an unusually excruciating form of cramp which affects inaccessible nether regions. Destroys all concentration and is a particular pest to tight-rope walkers and brain surgeons. Said to be responsible for the massacre of the Light Brigade.

The Sebastopol position helps – squatting on haunches in the corner of the bedroom with eyes tightly closed and beads of perspiration on the brow. This usually works by daybreak but can cause alarm to the cleaning lady.

# Bad Breath

Some people are born great, some achieve greatness and some . . . well, some just have bad breath.

It varies in severity, but generally speaking, you know you're in trouble when you enter a room and people start climbing out of the windows.

Bad breath, it seems, has always been with us. Michelangelo's was reputably like that of a bison with a hangover. Contemporary acounts vouchsafe the fact that he was capable of emptying the Uffizi Gallery in less than a minute.

A particularly foul period coincided with his work on the Sistine Chapel. Things got so bad that he was eventually banished to spend all his time on top of a ladder, where, as luck would have it, he got bored and started to do the ceiling.

It is now known that bad breath is nearly always caused by bacteria, which feed off bits of brussel sprout that get stuck between the teeth. Studies at Yale and Oxford have suggested that the solution might be to swallow them whole.

If you're careful, you can sometimes mask the effect at moments by turning your head to one side. This is largely unsatisfactory, as your partner may assume your sweet nothings are being directed at someone sitting behind her and, in any event, all you'll end up with is a stiff neck.

Another tip worth considering is avoiding any words beginning with a letter likely to cause a problem. This is where a speech therapist can be very useful. Thus, 'Samantha, Samantha, suck my nostrils', might be replaced by 'Why don't we go to the pub?'

# Frostbite

Frostbite is nature's way of telling you not to take a family holiday on the east coast, which in any case has been ruined since the SAS have started to use it as a punishment camp.

Here are some general tips:

1. When sunbathing, wear at least six layers of clothing.
2. When returning to camp, get into the habit of counting toes.
3. If you must go on a picnic, make sure you're all roped together.
4. Never attempt to go out without seeking advice from your local Sherpa guide. Sherpas often visit Skegness and Cromer on adventure holidays.
5. Don't forget to take a llama.

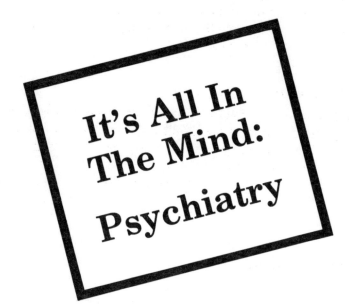

# It's All In The Mind: Psychiatry

The world of psychiatric problems is probably the most difficult of all the many disciplines that doctor has to encounter, with no rashes or spots to help him in his diagnosis.

You can do a lot to help by diagnosing your own problems.

Here are a few examples:

## Psychopaths

A psychopath is an individual with a faulty personality, characterised by anti-social behaviour, shiftlessness, lack of conscience and an inability to feel concern over anyone but himself.

A recent survey disclosed that, apart from politicians, there are over twenty thousand people with an overtly psychopathic tendency living in this country. A worrying feature was that they all meet together on Saturday afternoons to watch Chelsea.

## Inferiority Complex

Sadly, a lot of people simply hold themselves in very low esteem. They wander about, getting terribly introverted and generally presenting a hang-dog expression to the world. The trouble is, this behaviour brings out the very worst in people. They sense that there is a weaker member of the tribe in their midst.

Hence, our sufferer might be wandering about the streets, thinking how *awful* and *inadequate* he is, when a total stranger comes over and starts to beat him over the head, screaming 'Why are you so *inadequate*? God, I'm glad *I'm* not like you!'

This is obviously a difficult one to treat. Sometimes it's best to advise the sufferer that he *is* inadequate and to stop provoking people by staying indoors.

## Narcissism

In a way, this is the reverse of having an inferiority complex. Narcissists tend to swan around, stopping at every shop window in order to catch a glimpse of the Divine Creation reflected in the glass. They often carry around a small hand mirror to take an occasional peep when they've run out of shops.

Thankfully, these people are often run over by a bus while combing their hair.

## Paranoia

Some people spend their lives imagining that the whole world is after them. Typically, it manifests itself in people of a sensitive and vulnerable nature, such as ageing Germans, quietly living out their lives in Panama and Peru. Often associated with a reluctance to travel.

## Social Workers

Every field of human activity produces its hangers-on and if, for example, you're going around behaving like a loon, I'm afraid you're going to cop your fair share of social workers.

They are fairly typical in their appearance, arriving at your door in woolly stockings and sporting a beard. The trouble is that it's usually ages before they hold a case conference to decide what to do, by which time their problem's usually solved because you've moved to another area.

## Apathy

Apathy can be defined as want of feeling, passion or interest in anything. This can be a wonderful feeling when it comes to having to get out of bed or taking out the rubbish. The problem starts when you begin to feel the same about using toilet paper.

## Feeling Depressed?

If you find, say, that you've lost your job, your house has burnt down, your wife or husband has run off with another man – and you've got tapeworm – this can be extremely annoying.

If all these things happen to you in the same week, the chances are that by the Friday, you'll be feeling a little bit down about things.

At times like this, a visit to the doctor is most helpful, for with his wealth of experience, he'll be able to tell you that you're Depressed. He will then give you some green and yellow pills, or possibly some pink ones, and tell you to go away.

If this doesn't work, he'll put aside some special time to get down to the real nitty-gritty. During this frank exchange, he will take a full social, occupational, familiar and psychological history.

When your three minutes is up, he'll shake his head and solve both his and your problem by referring you to a Specialist.

There is often a three-to-eight-year waiting list to see the specialist, since it takes him an awfully long time to cure people, so that there's usually a considerable back-log. The other reason is that specialists in this field should ideally be sixty-to-seventy-year-old Middle European emigrés and nowadays, quite frankly, you just can't get them.

When you finally get to see him, he will ask you what the problem is. You will tell him, for example, that you feel you are not a whole person. He will nod and ask you whether, as a child, you liked to play with your faeces. Do not be alarmed. This is called Psychoanalysis.

Now this brings us to the first problem when dealing with psychoanalysts. As we have just seen, you give him a perfectly straightforward description of how you are feeling and he accuses you of doing something terrible with your poohs. What conclusions should one draw from this strange rejoinder? There are but two: either it is a profoundly insightful question designed to bring out a deeply held and long-forgotten truth, *or* he, too, is bonkers and quite possibly a pervert. So the first rule in choosing your analyst must always be: *Make sure he's not bonkers.*

## The history of psychoanalysis

The birth of psychoanalysis presents a fascinating story. It can be traced to a group of erstwhile Viennese layabouts, called Krösby, Nasch, Freud and Jung.

Much to their parents' disgust, they went off and formed a pop group, calling themselves, 'Jung, Gifted and Jewish'. They really weren't very good – the long, repetitive guitar riffs and distorted feedback finding little echo with the Austrian aristocracy of the 1890s.

Since Freud wrote most of the songs and Jung arranged the gigs, they started to copy most of the stick. Relations within the group became very strained, until inevitably the whole thing fell apart, with Krösby and Nasch finally emigrating to America in order to discover themselves and never being heard of again.

This left Freud and Jung in a quandary, for apart from anything else, their former colleagues had gone off with all the gear, leaving them with just a washboard, triangle and a pair of battered old phallic cymbals.

They soldiered on, with little success and diminishing conviction. Things finally reached a turning point after a disastrous appearance at the Salzburg Festival Fringe. They sold their instruments for scrap and started to thumb a lift back to Vienna.

During the journey, Jung, seated on the horse behind Freud, whispered something in his ear that was to change the course and complexion of medical history.

'Siggy,' he whispered, 'I want to tell you something.'

'What is it already?' replied Freud, coming out of a trance-like state induced by the horse's spine jogging up and down between his legs.

'I had a funny dream last night . . .' continued Jung. Freud cast his eyes to the heavens and tried to concentrate again on the horse's backbone.

' . . . It was about three nuns and a donkey.'

Freud snapped out of his kinetic pleasurings as if hit by a thunderbolt. Could this dream, this terrible dream, have a hidden and primordial meaning? Was this Jung's subconscious reaching out, begging to be grasped and understood? Above all, he wondered, did this mean that his friend of so many years harboured secret desires to be a zoo-keeper in a convent?

Thus did Sigmund Freud give birth to psychoanalysis on the back of a horse.

From that moment, they worked like men possessed – writing, lecturing, researching. They established beyond peradventure the unhealthy relationship between Jewish mothers and their sons, and it was no surprise when 'Kosher Encounters of the Wrong Kind' became a best-seller.

Ironically, this very fame spelt doom to their long and close friendship. Jung began to resent the fact that Freud was always discovering things just before he did. A traumatic realisation of this came to Jung while on a visit to England. On being presented to the Dowager of Stanhope, he greeted her with a curious, 'I must say, your Highness, that your breasts are looking wonderful'. Having been manhandled out of her Highness's presence, he was further infuriated to be told by a gleeful Freud that Jung's outburst was a perfect example of the Freudian Slip, which he'd just invented. Jung responded with a hefty kick in the groin and informed Freud that he'd just invented the Jungian Nutcruncher.

They never spoke again.

Freud went from strength to strength. 'Totem and Taboo' – a raunchy account of Red Indian Sexual Rites – sold out in two days, and a tantalising peep at something called 'The Id' is mentioned in his later works. No one is actually sure to this day what the Id is, and indeed doubt whether it actually exists. Many believe it to be merely another ploy used by a mischievous Freud to infuriate Jung, who probably spent many fruitless years trying to find it.

## Other Forms of Treatment

### Group Therapy

When psychiatrists get really busy, they tend to panic. There's nothing more disconcerting than to treat someone who thinks he's Napoleon, when Attila the Hun is wrecking the waiting-room because he thinks you're spending too much time on Napoleon.

This is where Group Therapy is so useful. The psychiatrist can then get a job lot in and do them all in one go. This is also popular with the patients, as they can often get the 'party rate' and save a few bob.

So what exactly goes on during group therapy? The general idea is that everyone sits round in a circle and by talking through and sharing their experiences, they can help themselves to come to terms with their problems.

In practice, what usually happens is that nobody talks until the last two minutes, when fighting breaks out. This is known as 'inter-relating'.

Normally, there is quite a waiting-list to get a seat on these sessions. So do look out for the late cancellation, if necessary using a bucket shop. They can often get you in on a charter group as long as you book three weeks in advance and don't mind sharing the session with people who come from Luton. Be sure to get there early in order to claim your seat. The psychiatrist will often put out one too few chairs just to get things festering nicely.

### Confrontational Therapy

This is an offshoot of group therapy and is used for really difficult cases. The participants take off all their clothes and proceed to yell and scream abuse at one another for an hour. When the bell goes, they put their clothes back on and go home. It really does seem to work, although difficulties can arise if the patient misses a week. He tends to get acute withdrawal sysmptoms, only finding relief by taking off all his clothes and yelling abuse, etc. This obviously has its drawbacks if, at the time, you're shopping in Harrods or singing in a choir.

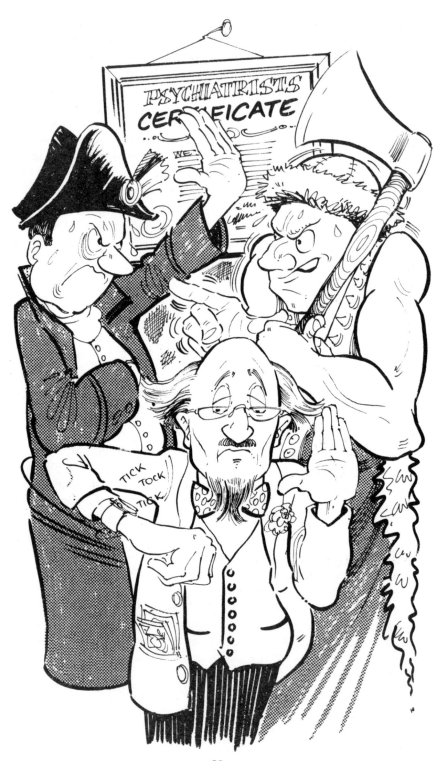

## Behaviour Therapy

This is designed to iron out defects in everyday living. By careful counselling, a patient can be weaned off what some might think is unsocial behaviour, like biting the heads off frogs.    It often works on a system of small rewards. With impotence, for example, the male is made to run down a passage. When, at a given moment, someone rings a bell and he manages an erection, he is rewarded with a piece of cheese. This is an example of the Pavlovian Response, so called because the original reward used was a mixture of fruit and meringue. This pattern is soon learnt by the male. All his wife or partner then has to do is to keep a ready supply of Roquefort handy for those rainy afternoons when the children are out, always remembering never to leave him alone anywhere near the delicatessen cheese counter where he could overdose and cause a lot of damage to himself and the shop-fittings.

# Phobias

The true place of behaviour therapy, however, is in the treatment of Phobias.

A phobia is an essentially morbid, exaggerated and irrational hatred of something. Here are a few to dream about.

## Spider Phobia

The treatment given to victims of spider terror illustrates perfectly how behaviour therapy works.

The sufferer is seated in an empty bath and a minute member of the spider family is allowed to crawl up through the plughole. The staff then withdraw, leaving the patient in the bath to freak. Now comes the clever bit. Over a period of weeks, the patient is placed in the same bath and, gradually, larger and hairier spiders crawl in up the plughole. It is extraordinary to watch the results. Within an amazingly short period of time, the same person, who was a gibbering wreck with a spider the size of a pinhead, can now sit naked in the bath in the company of a massive and revolting bird-eating monster, positively screaming the place down.

## Dental Phobia

No one actually likes going to the dentist, but some people have built up such a terror of it that they'd prefer to be . . . well, in a bath full of bird-eating spiders.

Again, behaviour therapy can be of great help. Using the same principle, the panic-stricken patient is first introduced to an easy-going, good-looking chap who engages her in conversation about this and that, just to break the ice. After a few minutes, he'll say something like, 'Oh, by the way, I'm a dentist'. Perhaps that is all that will be attempted on the first visit.

On subsequent occasions, 'Paul', (that won't be his real name) might mention that he really does find her terribly attractive and nice to talk to and 'By the way, I'd really like to have a look at those teeth'. The phobee is thus won over and, before she knows it, she is lying back to allow this wonderful person to give her a full examination.

By the third or fourth visit, 'Paul' will whisper to her something along the lines of, 'God, you've got beautiful teeth. I'd really like to have a go at them. How about this little one just over here?' She will allow him to do it, realising that for the first time she has allowed a dentist to place his finger in her mouth.

By visit five or six, she will happily lie back and allow him to do practically anything he wants. This is the 'moment critique'. ' . . . I call this my drill,' murmurs Paul. To the howl of the air-turbine and the smell of burning dentine, the relationship is consummated and the patient, once so terrified, will be coming back for weekly fillings.

## Francophobia

Until quite recently, the above condition wasn't even considered to be a phobia at all, inasmuch as it was a healthy and quite rational dislike of a race of people who professed not to speak English.

Of course, all that changed as we were hustled into the EEC when some bureaucratic twerp in Brussels decided it was time to stop being beastly to the Frogs.

Did Trafalgar and Waterloo mean nothing at all? Were we being asked to renege on hundreds of years of great British tradition? Indeed we were.

To the man in the street, all this was of little import, but denizens of the Foreign Office and Diplomatic Corps suddenly found themselves obliged to attend compulsory Francophobia Aversion Therapy Clinics in a special building just off Old Compton Street.

Wincing under-secretaries entered the building to be greeted by endless portraits of de Gaulle and the faint smell of garlic. The discordant sounds of Debussy harried the unfortunate gents as they hurried to their classroom, where mornings were spent getting through a packet of Gauloise and watching re-runs of old Jean-Paul Belmondo films.

Frogs' legs and snails were, of course, *de rigueur* at lunchtime, and were crunched to the dulcet tones of the revered Charles Aznavour and hitherto totally reliable chaps could be seen dining at the local brasserie, enjoying a joke, *in French*, with the unmentionably unctuous *Maître d'*.

Of course, it wasn't long before the people who matter decided that enough was enough and met secretly to halt the process. They came up with a programme of Reversion Therapy, where the victims were weaned off the worst of the pernicious gallic affliction and were reintroduced to the more traditional British values such as fast food, warm beer and Charlton Athletic.

## Claustrophobia and Agorophobia

Perhaps the less said about this pair the better, because therapists are always forgetting which one is which, so that unfortunate claustrophobies are usually stuck in locked lifts while agorophobies are sent off on rambling holidays in the Pyrenees. Still, no one's perfect.

## Aversion Therapy

Aversion Therapy consists of replacing something you like with something you don't like, so that every time you feel like doing it, you won't like it. It can be a bit of a killjoy, as I feel it's often best to have a go and worry about the mess afterwards, but that's just a personal opinion.

This therapy is really reserved for recidivists and hard- liners and generally consists of being given electric shocks to stop you doing something wicked or merely unhealthy.

Using the adage 'You've got to be cruel to be kind', recalcitrant nose-pickers, for example, are often wired up to the mains. This doesn't always break them of the habit, but at least forces them to pay a higher price for their pleasures.

# Dreams

Whole books have been written on this subject, but because bookshop owners unaccountably put them on their top shelf, often sandwiched between 'photographing the Nude' and 'Polynesium

Sex Rituals', they are often stared at, but rarely taken down.
Dreams roughly fall into the following categories:

*a* Those you can talk about –
e.g. Wanting to be Queen and playing for Sheffield Wednesday.
*b* Those you'd prefer not to talk about –
e.g. Wanting to be Queen and playing for Arsenal.

| *Dream* | *Probable Meaning/Advice* |
|---|---|
| **1** Robert Redford's got the hots for you. | This is bad news for clergymen and lumberjacks. Often caused by falling asleep in an unnatural position. |
| **2** You are Attila the Hun and are marauding through Europe. | You're in need of a break. What about that package holiday to Benidorm you promised the family? |
| **3** Trains going into tunnels. | Often inspired by the fear that your wife is having an affair with a baggage handler at King's Cross Station. Strangely, men have been having this dream years before trains were invented. |
| **4** An overpowering sensation that you want to spend a penny. | You've just spent one and ninepence. Best to change the sheets and consult a urologist. |
| **5** You've just become manager of Arsenal. | It's your subconscious having a joke. Often associated with a morbid fear that people are laughing at you. |
| **6** You've just become manager of Fulham. | People *are* laughing at you. |

**7** You imagine you are a doctor and there are ninety-eight angry people waiting to be seen.

You *are* a doctor and you've overslept by an hour and a quarter.

**8** You imagine you are being punched, elbowed and kicked from a point high up on your back, across your buttocks and down your legs.

You've been snoring.

**9** As above, but the blows are more indiscriminate.

You've got dreadfully drunk and got into bed with your girl-friend's husband.

**10** You've got into bed with your girl-friend's husband.

He must be an absolute smasher.

**11** You've just scored a barn-storming century on your debut for England, but feel strangely uncomfortable.

You're still wearing your box.

**12** You are an English tennis player and you've just won Wimbledon.

You're going insane.

**13** A repetitive dream that you want to be Pope.

You're Jewish and in a bit of a rut.

**14** You've just been elected Pope.

You're Jewish with very good connections.

**15** North Sea Oil is just about to run out and you discover how to convert base metals into gold.

You're Nigel Lawson. Try not to wake up.

**16** You are a pathetic little wimp who keeps on getting beaten up by the leader of the gang.

You are a senior government minister. It's your subconscious telling you not to be put upon. Stand up and say what's on your mind and be rewarded with a quiet life on the back benches.

**17** You are making mad and passionate love to Bo Derek and Madonna.

Assuming that don't actually have the acquaintance of these ladies, this type of dream is usually caused by an inappropriate physical manifestation that occasionally happens to men just before dawn. It is quite normal and usually goes away of its own accord by the time you get to the office.

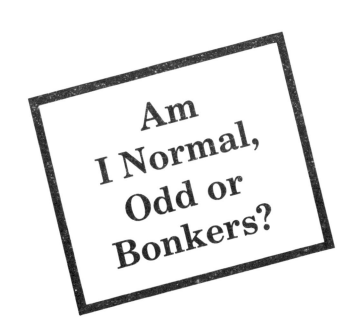

# Am I Normal, Odd or Bonkers?

Throughout the ages, people, some of them quite famous, have behaved in strange ways.

Pope George III, for example, puzzled the assembled thousands in St Peter's Square by prancing around the balcony pretending to be a kangaroo.

And was it not Bonar Law who enlivened dull debates in the House of Commons by dangling his naked buttocks over the front benches, exclaiming, 'May I have the pleasure of the next dance Milady?'

These people were certifiably and quite plainly bananas. But what about you? Is your behaviour normal, odd or are you indeed *bonkers*?

The following is called a Cuckoo Grid and will help you decide for yourself.

| | *Normal* | *Odd* | *Bonkers* |
|---|---|---|---|
| You're worried you left the back door open and come home to check. | You've gone next door for a cup of tea. | You're at your mother's funeral. | You're on holiday in Australia. |
| You are on your first free-fall parachute jump. | You become momentarily but severely incontinent. | You look round to admire the view, but for some reason you can't keep your eyes open. | You take the opportunity to catch up on some reading. |
| You are spending all your spare time teaching your pet bird to talk. | You are the owner of an adorable little budgie. | You are the owner of an adorable little budgie that unfortunately expired some-time ago after falling into the chip-frier. | You are the owner of a griffon vulture. |

| | | | |
|---|---|---|---|
| You always go on holiday to the same place. | You've been going back to Mrs Mason in Broadstairs every year since 1957. The food's excellent and the Masons are such lovely people. | You've been going back to France every year since 1957 because you find the French are such lovely people. | You've been going back to the Persian Gulf every year to spend a week or two on Kharg Island. The food's excellent and the Khomeinis are such lovely people. |
| You wake up and imagine you are a reincarnation of Alexander the Great. | You stay in bed and hope it goes away. | You keep it to yourself, but quietly change your name by deed poll. | You book a charter flight and invade Mesopotamia. |

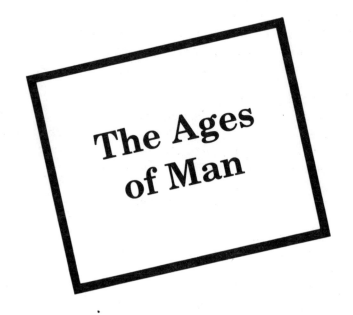

# The Ages of Man

# Childbirth

So much has already been written on this subject, that I feel reluctant to add to the confusion. I do feel, however, that a book of this kind should include a small chapter for the partner who, in the hurly-burly of confinement tends to be the bridesmaid – daddy.

## The early days

Morning sickness is a miserable experience. It usually happens to daddy soon after pregnancy has been confirmed and is normally caused by his having celebrated rather too well with the chaps in the pub. Try to be sympathetic and keep a bucket handy.

This generally goes after a few weeks, once the novelty has worn off, as does backache, which is experienced by daddy as a result of enforced over-exertion when mummy first decided she wanted to get pregnant.

On the subject of sex, may I have a little word with mums at this stage?

You will find that as your pregnancy progresses, daddy's desire for intercourse will tend to diminish. I cannot emphasise too strongly that this is quite normal. This is the period when daddy's hormones are preparing his body to undergo that wonderful change that comes when he starts to build his nest. Try to be gentle and understanding, and realise that his reticence is usually due to the discomfort he feels during the night because you are taking up more and more room in the bed. *Never, never* force anything on him he doesn't want, but if you feel your sexual demands must be met, try to adopt a position which won't take too much out of him and preferably without waking him up.

## The middle months

As your pregnancy progresses, so you will notice great physical changes taking place with daddy's body. His abdomen will get larger due to all the junk food he's now forced to eat because you're too tired to cook. He will tend to slouch around the house in his slippers. Climbing the stairs will become a major under-taking, with many stops on the way. You may be feeling tired as well, but try to encourage him by standing at the top of the stairs with a drink and some peanuts.

In general terms, then, daddy will think of himself as a bit of a frump. Psychologically, this represents a dangerous period. Try to encourage him to think positively. Encourage him to wear clothes from the Demis Roussos collection. Never be too tired and obsessed about your coming confinement to let daddy know just how *fabulous* you think he looks.

## The final days

A few days before confinement is due to take place, the hospital will often hold a 'father's night'. Daddy will be fairly immobile by this stage, but do take him along because it is designed to help the staff decide how best to look after him during the period of the birth.

This is a good time for *you* as well, because while he's out of the way, you can take the opportunity of familiarising yourself with the unit and what goes on there. Ask the staff to show you the instruments they'll use in delivering baby. Some mums seem to develop quite a phobia about these implements and what they do, and it is surprising how easily their minds are put to rest when they are shown the various prongs, rakes, wrenches and strimmers generally used for the job. Meanwhile, they'll have been working on daddy as well, by showing him what a nappy looks like and playing tape-recordings of a baby crying.

## Labour

You will first realise that labour has begun when you have your first contraction and daddy starts to whimper. It is very important that he is made to calm down, for there is a long way to go. During the early phase, there is no reason why you shouldn't potter around and generally distract him.

Why not make him a few sandwiches for the hospital? Or even better, check his little travelling case to make sure you've packed everything, especially a change of underwear.

Problems increase as the contractions become more severe. On no account start wailing, or you will have a full-blown panic on your hands from you know who. A good idea, every time you feel one coming on, is to mask your cries of pain by bursting into song with something from 'Seven Brides for Seven Brothers', or 'The Sound of Music'. This might alarm him, but muttering something about 'The Show' will jog his memory and get him sufficiently confused to keep him quiet.

The time will finally come, however, when you have to make a move to leave for the hospital. It is difficult to say exactly at what point this should be, but when daddy has got so beside himself with blind panic that he breaks his waters, then it's generally time to go.

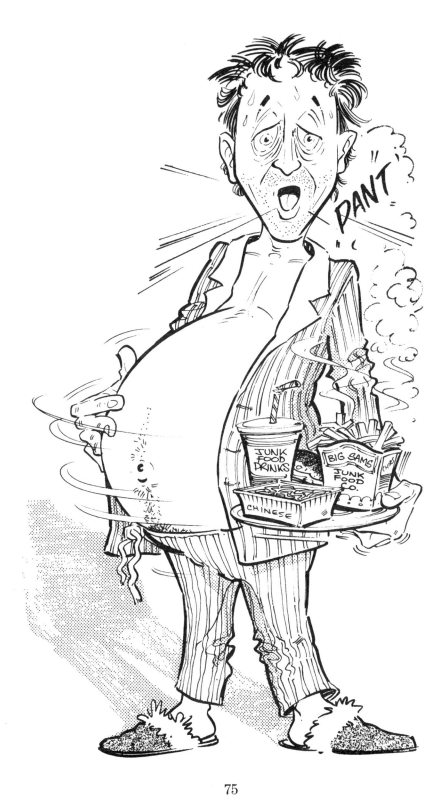

## The hospital

As you reach the hospital, there might be a final protest from Rambo to the effect of 'I'm not coming in'. He doesn't really mean this and a curt but firm reply of 'Well you just stay out here while I have the baby' will usually be sufficient to call his bluff and he'll follow you in, perhaps kicking the door as he does so.

When you get to the delivery unit, you will be given your own room. Park daddy on a chair and tell him not to move. This should be the last you'll hear from him, although he'll remain a bit of a grump throughout when he realises he really isn't going to get much attention.

Now, what about you? Start taking in your surroundings. Delivery rooms are generally a veritable hive of activity, with nurses and midwives attending busily to their work. You settle back for the long wait, only to become aware that the impression of calm and efficiency is somewhat spoilt by a familiar-looking male trying to look inconspicuous. But his grey pallor, sweating palms and general impression of terror tell you who it must be – the doctor.

The hours will pass slowly. Contractions will come more frequently now and increase in their severity. When things get too much, concentrate on your breathing exercises and use the gas and air mask, if you can get it off daddy.

In the later stages, the room may well be rent by loud shrieks of torment, as daddy tries a few attention-seeking attacks. Give him back the gas-mask and tell him to shut up.

Eventually, the magic moment will arrive. A final heave, and daddy will be violently sick.

As baby starts to emerge, the delivery team will get hysterical, with everyone screaming, 'It's coming. Bloody hell, it's coming.' With a slurp that sounds like a large bath emptying, baby is born. Someone will then give it a slap. Don't be alarmed, it's just to stop it crying.

Very soon afterwards, another bit comes out. Again, don't worry, it's not another baby, but the afterbirth.

When all the action is over and the walls have been hosed down, a remarkable transformation will be seen in daddy. He'll hold baby in his arms and croon away, as if he's just done all the work. Resist the temptation to kick him because you will need to conserve all your energy.

One final word of warning. Another temptation in the euphoria of the moment is to name your baby after nurse. Be careful, she might be called Lucrezia or Zenobia . . . .

## Should I Breast Feed?

I would hesitate to make any hard and fast rules for this most vexatious subject, except just to mention that it should ideally be one of mummy's jobs. This has a great stabilising influence on the marriage, inasmuch as parents will no longer have rows in the middle of the night about whose turn it is to get up and do the feeding.

Daddies, on the whole, think that breast-feeding is a wonderful invention and will generally mutter as much at 3.45 a.m., before sinking back into comatosed bliss.

Now mums, of course, become absolutely exhausted during this period. Although broken nights and lack of sleep play a part, the main reason is undoubtedly the fact that they have to spend all their time lugging around such a whopping great pair of milkers.

Should one breast-feed in public? If you want to be considered a right-on, laid-back and politically-sound mother, there can, indeed, only be one answer. Indeed, a lot of women who read the *Guardian* generally have babies just so they can heave out a whopper on the Piccadilly line during rush-hour. The fact that six other people have to give up their seats just doesn't seem to worry them.

## A Quiet Word for New Daddies

Since the birth of your child, you have probably been worrying and possibly shedding a tear or two about the sad state of your testicles. This is, I'm afraid, the heavy price you have to pay for the wear and tear involved in making a baby.

Once they were proudly spherical, lovingly tended and, had there been such competitions, would have had a rosette pinned on them. Now, wrinkled and tattered, saggy and useless, they just hang there, for all the world like a pair of pink prunes that have been left over from a long-forgotten pudding.

Look, I don't want to be a Jeremiah, but I'm a doctor and I can tell you that they've had it. Forget about silicone implants; they look extremely silly and you end up sitting on them the whole time. You can try wearing specially designed underpants with a system of supporting elastic, but really, the thing to do is to accept that they've had a good innings – you've got all the wear you're ever going to get out of them and above all, don't try to look at them too often. A sympathetic and loving wife can always be a great source of solace by not laughing whenever you drop your pants.

# Growing Up : Advice for Mums

Watching your child grow, learning new things and bringing joy and happiness into what is sometimes a drab world, is reward enough for all the work you have to do in making sure the precious little things grow up healthily.

Sometimes, however, things do go wrong and your child becomes poorly. What to do?

I feel that the treatment of their aches and pains can be divided into the following distinct age-groups:

a 0-22 years.
b 22 and over.

Since much has already been written about the younger child, I would like to concentrate on the latter group.

## The late developer

All too often I have worried mums coming to see me at the surgery with their eldest child, worried perhaps that he is not making the physical and emotional progress he should be. Typically, the child might be a bed-wetting accountant or maybe a prospective member of parliament who's prone to attention-seeking attacks of prolonged vomiting at teatime.

Whatever the symptoms, the greatest caution must be exercised in dealing with such children. Generally, all they are seeking is a little self-assurance. Maybe that thumb-sucking you've been worried about is just his way of showing you that he's worried about something – perhaps that approaching exam or by-election.

You must remember that your child is no longer 'your little baby' and is striving to reach out for manhood. Try to encourage him in this by eliminating things that might be holding back his advance towards maturity, like winding him after meals.

It will do wonders for the confidence and assurance of the late developer if you can get him off breast-feeding. This, of course, is easier said than done, because, my goodness, over the years they do get a taste for it; but when he comes back from the office for his midday feed, see if you can gently introduce him to bits of mashed banana and tinned prunes. Within days he'll be toddling back to work with a satchel full of tins of egg yolk and bone broth.

## Sleepy problems

The late developer will often be a problem at bedtime. This is

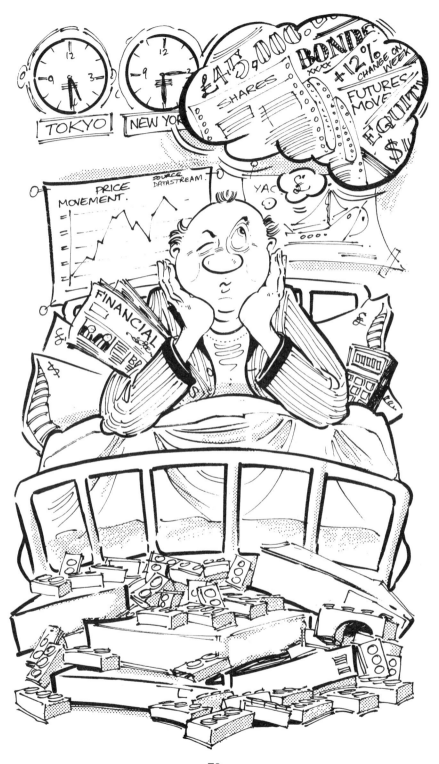

hardly surprising, for his mind is chock-a-block full of new and sometimes contradictory discoveries.

Just imagine it. Your little boy has got himself a job in the Futures Market, earning in excess of £45,000 a year before bonuses and all he wants to do is buy more Lego.

Try, therefore, to avoid over-stimulation just before bedtime. Less romping games and more quiet encouragement in the shape of subdued bedtime stories along the lines of: 'Think how much money you're going to earn tomorrow!' or 'You remember that nice boat you wanted? Well, mummy and daddy will take you down to the Boat Show and get it for you!'

Kiss him goodnight, tuck him in, leave him with a copy of the *FT* and a pocket calculator and you won't hear another peep out of him as he drifts off to bo-bo's, dreaming of Rio Tinto Zinc.

## Temper tantrums

This, of course, can cause great embarrassment to parents. Its onset is characterised by the child flinging himself on to the ground, screaming and kicking, and might be climaxed by him biting either himself, yourself, a piece of furniture, a passing stranger or a policeman. This is particularly difficult to handle if you happen to be in a supermarket and your child is approaching thirty.

What lies behind this distressing behaviour?

Don't forget that your child is discovering new things every day. His own desk at the office perhaps, or a new girl-friend; it could be any of these and more. The important point to understand is that he's trying to show you that he's ready to throw off the protective mantle of childhood. Your little boy is growing up! So encourage him with words like, 'You clever baby! Mummy understands that you're just doing this to show me you're ready to become a man! You just lie there and mummy will come back with some sweeties for my *brave, big, grown-up* baby!'

If this doesn't work, kick him until he gets up.

## Discovering his woogie

It is often about this age, when everything else seems to be going to plan, that he first discovers his penis. This is a particularly difficult time and potentially dangerous, especially if it coincides with a temper tantrum (see previous section).

Of course, having discovered it, he won't be able to leave it alone, probably showing it to everyone at the office.

The first thing is to reassure worried mums that it is perfectly normal, being the natural curiosity of the late developer discovering a part of his body that he had hitherto probably dismissed as a bit of gristle. He now finds, however, that during moments of stress, such as important meetings, etc., he can gain much solace by merely holding it. In other words, it has become his comforter and, apart from anything else, is much the most convenient because it can never cause panic by being left anywhere.

The psychological importance of his comforter should not be lost on the caring and discerning mother. Never, never say anything like, 'Roger, stop playing with your bonker!' or worse, warning him that his hair will fall out if he doesn't. Rather let him get over it in his own good time, knowing that as he matures he'll probably find other uses for it anyway.

Until that time, encourage him to think of it as something rather special. Why not give it a name? I don't mean like 'Cecil' or 'Piers', but a familiar and reassuring one like 'Woogie'.

One day, your patience and understanding will be rewarded when he comes home and announces that he's discovered that girls don't have Woogies and wants to know what a Boogie is.

After that, he'll probably leave home and cram in twenty years of Boogie-Woogie in a week.

## Adolescence

Adolescence is such a wonderful time for growing boys and girls. Above all, it is a time for discovering things – delinquency, acne and periods being the most common.

As parents, you suddenly find that, almost overnight, no longer are they your little babies, but rapidly changing and maturing adults, with apparently undesirable habits and anti-social tendencies. You will find these very distressing and difficult to comprehend. But you must resist the temptation to criticise just because they're different. Try to remember that social mores change. Just as you were probably brought up on a diet of sex, drugs and rock and roll, they want to show their independence by organising pop concerts to feed the Third World. *This doesn't mean it's wrong.* The point to realise is that *they'll soon get over it* and become sensible adults like you and me.

The key to maintaining a stable relationship with one's teenagers is to try to be their *friends*. Spend a little time with them. For instance, when your boy brings back his girl-friend for the first time, don't just leave them all alone in the sitting room –

make a point of going in there. Sit on the sofa with them, put a friendly arm around the pair of them and have a good old *chat*. Make a special effort to get to know the girl-friend. It's amazing how a few questions like, 'And what are you going to do when you're a little older, poppet?', accompanied by a reassuring squeeze on the arm, will totally put her at ease. And your boy will be so proud of you, especially when she tells him she thinks you're a real gas.

Your daughter's boy-friends need somewhat different treatment. Make your intentions clear from the outset by never leaving them together in a room. You don't even have to sit down with them. Merely standing there, either just staring at them or looking out of the window, will be sufficient to reassure your beautiful daughter that you are not going to let a ponce with an ear-ring take any advantage. She may never mention it the next day, but you can be sure that her silence at the breakfast table hides the over-powering feelings she now has for you.

## The Middle Years

A time to enjoy the fruits of one's labours. You have survived the plagues of puberty, the bottomles pit of adolescence, the ravages of the rat race and the ignominies of rubbing groins with the mob in the debasing scrummage for a mate in life. No more schooldays being lashed round sodden playing fields in PE kit. No more sordid Friday nights clutching a beaker of stale Beaujolais on some puke-ridden staircase with a hundred other spotty Herberts. You've flogged your old Kinks records, you've flogged your rugby shirt and you've given the *Karma Sutra* to Oxfam. And good riddance. Smile. Go and mow the lawn, you fat frump – for Yours is the Kingdom of Heaven.

### Discovering Yourself

Few experiences in life match the warm glow of gazing upon one's own insurpassable beauty in the mirror. Seduced by old familiar landmarks, it takes but a small hurdle of self-deception to see still the fresh eager face of our youth staring back at us like the same spring rosebud that only yesterday braced itself against life's April showers. The sparkling, slightly uncertain eyes; the milk and honey smoothness of that brow; that cheek – verily the grey shadow of age has barely caressed them.

Comforted by this living proof of eternal youth, the wise virgin now creeps softly from the bathroom before wakefulness ensues and the full white light of morning floods in. Though to tarry may be tempting, to linger too long before this vision of loveliness risks weakening its spell. Remember, 'whom the Gods wish to destroy, they first make pretty'. Don't waste vain seconds pouting those full girlish lips; finish shaving and go serenely about your business. Do *not* stand admiring your whippy hips. Do *not* examine your tongue.

For those who do such things will one day see a new and unfamiliar image metamorphosing through the condensation. Across the no-man's land of tooth-mugs and deodorant sticks, ignoring the choking mists of aftershave, through the steam the reflection of the beast bears lewdly down on you. Awful . . . Naked . . . It is the *enemy*. It is *you*.

## Self Pity
At this terrible moment in one's life it is understandable to feel bitter. You have, after all, just discovered that what you believed to be the embodiment of beauty is really rather unsightly. Transfixed by the new knowledge of your shapelessness, you search vainly for bits that still possess vestiges of youth or at least have a certain old-world charm. Patiently lifting folds of skin may sometimes reveal previously undiscovered areas of outstanding natural beauty. Sadly, it is more likely to uncover further unspeakable horrors such as yeast colonies or skin tags.

## Coming to Terms
The first rule of accepting lost youth is not to get too depressed about it. Accept your new persona with pride and dignity. Burn all your old photograph albums of the school PE display and think positively about the acquisition of wisdom, experience and obesity. Don't ruminate pointlessly about being only thirty-one. If you still think life isn't worth living and want to top yourself, don't go in for anything messy involving high buildings or trams. Just because life has dealt you an unkind trick, there is no need to go upsetting your doctor who may well be trying to par the four-teenth hole when news of your emulsification reaches him.

## Fighting Back
A careful programme of rehabilitation can soon have you feeling like a lissom eighteen-year-old. Forget it. No lissom eighteen-year-old is going to look at you until you've shed several of those pallid doughy folds of blubber and started the fight back to fitness.

Unfortunately, this is going to involve an unpleasant process known medically as exercise.

**Starting**

The first rule is to remember your limitations. Don't forget you have spent the last decade or two slumped in various chairs – at the office, in the home, in the car, on the lavatory. Sudden bursts of energy could well shoot off a clot. Start from strength. Your hands are probably still in reasonable condition from moving biros about, dialing telephone numbers and changing the television channels. This is a useful springboard to build from. Try crushing tangerines in your fists and progress gradually to cricket balls.

**Later**

Physical jerks. Don't be put off by your spouse sniggering. A few windmill exercises with the upper limbs will soon wipe the smile off, especially if you've had baked beans the night before. Above all, make it fun. Put some Val Doonican records on, swing those arms, brace those shoulders back and try to ignore the searing pain. Quick pause for breath, then running on the spot for two minutes; without breaking stride glide off smoothly into the bathroom, leap like a gazelle on to the bathroom scales and smash them to bits. Now try a press-up.

**Much later**

After some weeks the press-ups will seem almost effortless. You are now ready to advance to the skipping rope. Make sure you have plenty of room – ideally go outside. Avoid kitchens, delphiniums and garden ponds. If you choose the garden shed, be sure to move the lawnmower and, above all, the rake. Hold the two ends of the rope so that the loop rests gently against your calf muscles. Then, whip it swiftly over your head while at the same time heaving your colossal bulk off the floorboards for as long as seems reasonable. Beware of the so-called phalanx effect (named after the shield formation of Roman legions). In this phenomenon the hurtling rope scythes into your shins while you are in mid-air, lifting both legs high above the back of your head and causing an explosive rush of spittle. Impact with the ground is usually accompanied by an avalanche of garden implements and rupture of some less important internal organs.

## Jogging

You really must prepare sensibly for this. Remember that for the first few weeks you will almost certainly have to be brought home, perspiring and barely alive, by a taxi or sympathetic passer-by.

You don't want to look any more of a prat than you can possibly avoid. So go to a reputable sports dealer and get some kit that fits and doesn't cut off the blood supply if you swell up in the rain. Once you are on to two-mile runs, make sure your shorts are luminous in case you are out all night.

Beginners are advised to stay indoors at first. Build up from gentle jogs to the drinks cabinet to more demanding runs, yomping from the living room to an upstairs bedroom with a heavy briefcase full of sandwiches.

Once you have bought your gear you are committed. Your spouse will have told half the neighbourhood, and they are certain to have binoculars and vido equipment trained on your front door. Unless you enjoy humiliation, an early start is advisable, say 3 a.m. Go boldly and resolutely, striding out without a backward glance. Pace yourself carefully. Aim to make it to the end of the street, but as a precaution take a few letters in case you are conking out by the time you reach the pillar-box. You can always pretend you'd nipped out to post them.

## Perils of Jogging

Apart from the special problems of absolute beginners, other hazards await the gritty road runner.

**Gritty roads** can damage delicate, artistic feet. Fortunately, this shouldn't concern you in your present condition.

**Training Shoe Foot** is a fearful condition causing headache, vomiting and coma when training shoes are discovered in confined spaces such as toilets or picnic baskets.

**Acute Bollard Injury** is often found in accomplished runners who use Sony Walkmans. Collision is usually with a non-springy surface such as a concrete post and commonly occurs during haunting bits of Gershwin.

**Road Runners' Pit** is caused by multiple pile-ups of joggers in shopping precincts with stairwells. Can be very difficult to sort out. Rescuers should first disentangle loose items – shopping trolleys, old ladies and tins of cat food. Joggers should be disentangled one by one. Several may be shocked, minus their shorts or covered in yoghurt.

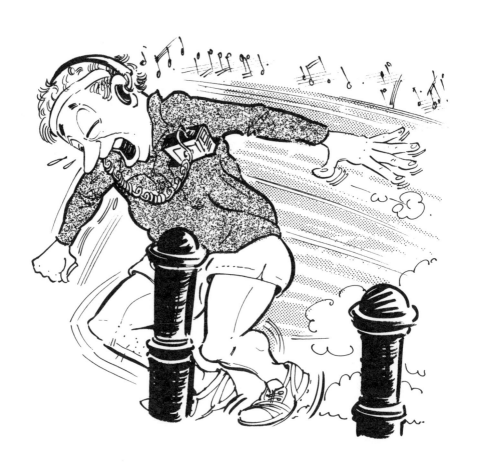

**Marathon Runners' Pit.** An infectious condition caught from unwholesome bed linen.

## Aerobics and Work-out Exercises

First invented by the Whirling Dervishes of the Khyber Pass before they discovered bridge. Aerobics was introduced into Western culture by Rommel as a means of building up stamina in his Panzer Divisions. Apparently abandoned after a particularly punishing session in a wild and an ugly bit of bitching about leotards, somehow this extraordinarily violent pastime has surfaced again. Sedate forms, practiced to Semprini music in some gentlemen's clubs, are probably not dangerous and may tone up the muscles supporting the liver. More energetic versions involve picking up your leg and whirling it round your head in time to disco music.

For the unfit this may be an ordeal, as some disco records last a minute and a half. The benefits are that victims are often able to catch up with all their paperwork during the prolonged recovery, and their trim waists and bunchy little bottoms are often the envy of the coronary care unit. Most bank managers, estate agents, etc. can get by without a bunchy little bottom. They should think carefully about aerobics and probably stick with less hazardous forms of exercise such as hang-gliding.

## Burn-out Syndrome

Typically affects career-minded, ambitious workaholics, often in the prime of their most productive years.
Warning signs:
*i* Arriving naked on the Tokyo Stock Exchange with a daffodil up the bum.
*ii* Trying to drive home in a filing cabinet.
*iii* Sitting under a running tap sucking a thumb and hugging a word processor.
By this time it's usually too late. Demise often follows the ingestion of large quantities of cordless telephones.

## Growth Movements

A cult introduced insidiously from California, spawned chiefly by psychogeriatrics in orange romper suits. There are numerous movements, most of which seem to involve taking all your clothes off and telling a crowd of total strangers what a miserable cur you are. I understand a lot of 'feeling' goes on (also conducted by total strangers) as well as quite a lot of shouting, running around and throwing up into buckets. I may not have covered all the points but, anyway, that's the gist of it.

## Growing Old

'You're only as old as you feel'. How often we've all heard that, fine old aphorism and how often we've felt like crowning the philosophising prat who first thought of it.

The point is, when *do* you start to get old? Some 55-year-olds feel and act as if they're 80, while some 80-year-olds feel and act as if they're 55. On the other hand, there are 80-year-olds who feel as if they're 107 and presumably 107-year-olds who don't feel a day over 102.

So how do you know you're getting old? Certainly, the acuity of your physical prowess will start to diminish. You might notice that your aim isn't as good as it used to be – on the golf course, for example, or having a wee.

In my experience, however, it is the person's reaction to his or her age that is the clue to age itself. For instance, a 10-year-old can't wait for his 11th birthday and indeed, wants to tell the world about it. On the other hand, a 40 or 50-year-old views the passing of each successive year with a mixture of resentment and dread, for although not yet old, he's getting there quicker than he bargained for. Moreover, he certainly doesn't want to talk about it.

A 60-year-old is quite simply depressed about the whole ghastly business.

But 70! You are reborn – a child again! And the next birthday can't come quickly enough, because then you can become an old bore about it, inviting complete strangers to guess your age, boasting of your grandchildren and basking in the glow of their admiration for what you can do at your age. But be prepared to meet your match in the person who tells you the truth and to shut you up mischievously hazards the guess that you look years older than you really are.

## Granny

Passing serenely into what has been charmingly called the 'Contemplative Age' is a precious and wonderful thing, and how right we are always to show and give the utmost respect to someone like Granny.

Granny, with her wealth of experience, panorama of knowledge and wisdom that can only come of a lifetime of tasting from life's sweet cup of understanding.

And isn't it the very least we can do to repay her in some small way by inviting her to come and live with us in the glory of her latter years? Oh, she'll protest. She'll be as stubborn as a mule because she is a fiercely independent woman. But finally, with a little cajoling, she'll take her rightful place in the very bosom of her family.

On the other hand, if, after a couple of weeks, you realise you've landed yourself with a meddling and bad-tempered old bat who's beginning to smell, you really must stick her in a home.

But where?

The short answer must be, I fear, as far away as possible. For instance, if you live, say, in Kent or Surrey, a good place to start looking might be the Cairngorms.

What sort of accommodation are we looking for? Well, the first question and indeed, at the end of the day, the *only* question of any relevance, must be, 'Is it secure?' Barbed wire, watch towers and patrolling Dobermans are by no means essential requirements for Old People's Homes, but it does give the rest of the family that certain extra little bit of peace of mind.

One thing that always preys on the mind after putting Granny on the train to her new home is Guilt.

'What have I done? Will she remember to change at Carlisle?' These feelings are quite normal and understandable. They can, however, become quite deep-seated and last for some days.

The clearest advice I can give to these poor people is never to forget, that thanks to modern communication, Granny is only a telephone call away. That doesn't mean you have to speak to her, but just remember that she's just a telephone call away.

One family of my acquaintance, who some might consider stony-hearted, sent their Granny on a world cruise. Nothing wrong with that, you might say, except they didn't tell her that it was only paid for up to Libya. All ended quite happily though; now a spry 97-year-old, she runs a small bordello just outside Tripoli.

## Living With Death

We all know we have to go sometime. Sooner or later we shall see the grim reaper himself wandering cheerily along the street or up the garden path waving a spare scythe. The first thing to cross your mind is probably, 'I wonder who he's come for?' Some while later the penny will drop that you've never actually *seen* him before, even though you've heard a lot about him. Not to worry.

Next thing will be you're out there helping him tidy up a few verges, thinking what a perfectly charming bloke he is. You won't worry about the wailing and gnashing of teeth back there. All that stuff about giving you a good send-off. Quite frankly, you'll wonder what all the fuss was about. Think of all the years you've been worrying about him coming – would you get everything done in time, have you provided for them all when you've popped it, would you have clean pants on? One thing about GR is he's extremely tolerant about the pants business. The only really annoying bit is everyone will be saying it's the way you would have wanted to go. I guarantee if you climbed into a sleeping bag full of jellyfish just as a steam roller thundered across your tent, someone would wipe a tear away and say 'At least he didn't suffer'.

## The River Styx

Not all things about the hereafter are total heresay. The River Styx, for example, possibly does exist. Legend suggests it's a black stretch of creepy water with a permanent greenish fog through which the grisly ferryman punts his way to collect you. He's got a cape and hood and all you can see are a pair of spooky yellow eyes. Actually, it's not a bit like this.

What happens is you queue up on the quayside of a rather inviting marina. Everyone's in straw boaters, and eating ice-creams and cracking jokes about being alive again. Occasionally someone will think of loved ones and burst into tears. This is a cue for everyone else to push him in and roar with laughter. It's really a lot of fun.

## Clothes

Somewhere along the way these all disappear. Nobody gives a monkey's about this.

## The Glass-bottomed Boat

This is the only sad bit, really. You go out in the boat and look through the glass at all your friends and loved ones asleep in their beds. Then you have cocoa and look at the stars. All in all, it's not as bad as going to the dentist.

## Euthanasia

This delicate subject is of course something of a taboo – Hippocratic oath and all that. Quite frankly, it's not like taking Fido to the vet just because his coat's lost its gloss. People would want to put each other down for all kinds of trivial reasons. In no time at all

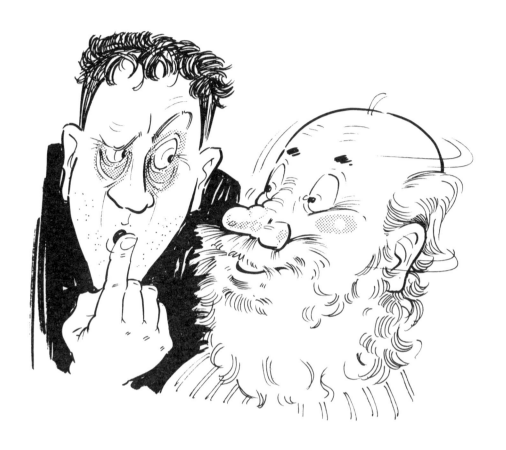

we'd live in a society which encouraged one to do the decent thing if you got a nasty sore throat or, perish the thought, you couldn't come up with the old jungle juice.

True, there are members of the aristocracy who proudly look forward to returning to their family vaults in the event of the balloon going up, so to speak. It's all perfectly painless. Off to the hotel of their choice for a slap-up meal and a bottle of Premier Grand Cru, then tossing themselves into the laundry chute. No hanging around moping. Not that I'm condoning such self-sacrifice. No indeed, where would civilisation be today if we all did that? One bottle of Retsina and Alexander the Great would have been flinging himself on to his sword. No Persian Empire. No Greek Empire. No British Empire.

Certain illegal organisations do, however, offer a range of services for those who want to dive into an early bath with a good splash. These are very variable, ranging from mere bucket shop knackers' yards to discreet and exclusive organisations like PURGE (Permanent Uninterrupted Rest for Gentlefolk.)

The better class of company stands head and shoulders above the run of the mill mail-order mercy killings merchants, offering an imaginative personalised service and many special offers.

Polynesian Paradise is a deluxe offer for those who've always wanted to perish in the sun-drenched South Pacific. Basically it's seven days on the beach in Tahiti, then they harpoon you and throw you to the crabs.

Rather expensive and wasteful, but terribly elegant, is the Yellow Roller. Not as horrid as it sounds, it's a gentle drive along the South Downs in a sparklingly smart Rolls Royce driven by a polite robot, then over Beachy Head with the engine purring at full throttle.

# Leisure and Work: Sport and Sports Medicine

As far as I'm concerned, anyone who spends his spare time chasing, kicking, jumping, hurling or even walking, needs to spend a serious length of time in the company of a shrink. Moreover, I have a strong feeling that if these people did an honest day's work, they wouldn't have any excess energy to burn up and would spend their spare time as I do, comfortably ensconced on a sofa, with the gas fire on max., before drifting off for an inter-meal bo-bo.

You may gather, therefore, that I consider all sporting pursuits unnecessary and hence any injury issuing therefrom self- inflicted and fully deserved, which is exactly what I tell groaning cricketers who come whining to my surgery after getting a ball in the nadgers.

## A Short History of Sport

I suppose it's fair to surmise that sports injuries started when cavemen started to toss the boulder. On the whole, though, there is little evidence to suggest that Neanderthal Man was ever really much of a sporty type, mainly due, it's thought, to the fact that point-to-point mammoth racing never really caught on.

What *did* catch on though, were the Christians being thrown to the lions. Although many consider it to have been a blood-sport, at least it combined people being chewed up with a love of wildlife – a lesson surely for us today.

In any event, the Romans and lions certainly enjoyed themselves, and the Christians, if they were honest, would probably have admitted to a sense of achievement in contributing to such a happy and popular spectacle.

More importantly, these events heralded the first appearance of the Trainer, although, to be honest, his ministrations were by necessity fairly brief and it has to be said that a quick application of the Magic Sponge and an encouraging pat on the behind were more symbolic than anything else.

So what, meanwhile, had been happening in this country? We had, in fact, entered a golden age, where virtually no sport was being played at all. True, the Romans did try and set up a Christians and Lions Club in what later became known as Dagenham, but this soon petered out through lack of interest, government money and Christians.

For the next 1,500 years or so, sport took a back-seat as people began to realise that they could get just as much enjoyment and exercise by starting wars with each other. Thus it was that expressions such as 'Groin-strain' and 'Hamstring Trouble' began to filter back from the Crusades while Edward III nearly missed the Battle of Crécy altogether because of a stubbed toe.

By the end of the nineteenth century, wars, although still popular in this country, had rather lost their appeal across the channel, mainly because the French had lost so many. Trafalgar and Waterloo were bad enough, but the Retreat from Moscow had made them very depressed and morose. A change of manager made absolutely no difference and they were becoming fairly desperate when the Baron de Camembert had a brilliant idea and invented the Olympic Games. This proved immensely popular as it gave the French something else to aim for, as well as providing multinational drugs companies with a healthy boost.

The Generals, not surprisingly, were fairly hacked off by all this, so a compromise was reached whereby the Games would be held every four years, with wars fitted in as and when time permitted – an arrangement that has stood the test of time.

The French were now happy, which, if nothing else, was a relief to the rest of Europe. They still didn't win anything, but didn't have to travel so far to get beaten.

Hence a new era was born. The British, meanwhile, had not been idle. They had exported not only Cricket but British Values to the very outposts of the Empire. Savage natives, who only years previously had been spending their leisure time by eating each other, were now playing the Noble Game, with far-flung fields resounding to cries of 'Well played Sir', as they settled down to a post-match beer, before tucking in to the twelfth man.

And so, sadly, we come to the present day, when you can't get to your car without being mown down by a gang of sweaty joggers, when hours of television are set aside to catch Terry Griffith advancing crab-like around the table to line up the final black and is only interrupted by something really urgent, like the Third World War or the lacrosse results. Incidentally, whatever happened to the honest-to-goodness and traditional World War? All we ever get now is World Cups.

It gives me the greatest pleasure, therefore, to enumerate the following and satisfyingly long list of Sporting Injuries.

## Athletics Injuries

### Fosbury Flop
Temporary impotence arising from unforeseen and traumatic collision with the high jump bar.

95

### Pole Vault
Quite severe injury can ensue when the pole slips during the ascent phase and gets stuck up the nostril.

### Shot Put
Newcomers to this discipline can end up with severely crushed toes.

### Hammer Throwing
One of the basic precepts of this event is not to forget to leave go as you throw it. Over-confident types who don't heed this warning can be flung up to 270 feet. You can also end up with extremely long arms.

### 100-Metre Sprint
Going like the clappers is one thing; being able to stop is another. Failure to do so can lead to writing yourself off. As you can also take a few dozen spectators with you, it is prudent to make sure you are adequately insured for third parties.

### Relay Races
Due to faulty change-over technique, the baton can become irretrievably lost up your waiting team-mate as he crouches expectantly waiting for you to wham it into his back-stretched grasp. Such being life, things can go wrong and the afore-mentioned baton can often only be extricated from your team-mate by the expert attention of a rectal surgeon.

### Javelin
The most unfortunate 'Kebab Disaster' can occur when two or more unwary track officials are skewered at a time.

### 50-Km Walk
Not so much physical injury as psychological trauma, resulting from inability to stop walking in any other way. Especially embarrassing when processing up the wedding aisle.

## Swimming Injuries
### Springboard Diving
Performing the almost legendary reverse triple somersault double loop flick-flack manoeuvre is fraught with dangers, none more so than the impact of the nose on the concrete of an empty swimming pool.

### Synchronised Swimming
This extremely silly sport cannot be considered dangerous but it is as well for protagonists to remember that unwanted pregnancy

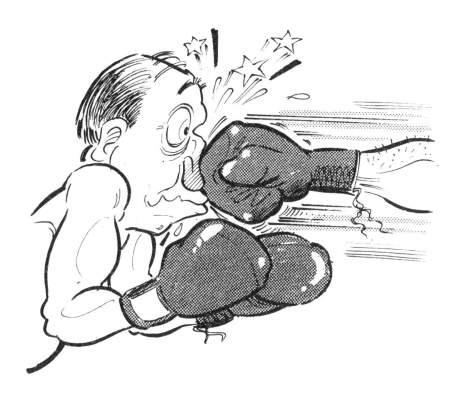

is an ever-present danger. Apart from this, loss of orientation can lead to mass-drowning, although this itself has become a major spectator sport on Japanese TV.

## Tennis Injuries
Nearly all injuries in this sport are suffered by the umpire. They are usually inflicted by psychotic Americans when they sense that the match is slipping away from them.

These include:

### Forehand
Usually delivered to the nose.

### Backhand
A surreptitious blow directed at the ear.

### The Rally
Rarely seen, but consists of a quickfire attack about the head by both players.

### Drop Volley
Gets its name from the effect of a stiff-armed jab in the groin with a racket handle.

### Tennis Elbow
The Americans consider this to be an art form. With correct timing, a well-aimed pointed elbow can land smack on the Adam's Apple.

### Smash
Considered the least subtle and most difficult to get away with.

The tennis authorities are starting to come down very hard on these offences and are handing out fines of up to £25, unless the player says he's not going to pay, in which case that's fair enough.

## Basketball Injuries
In a sport where anyone under 7 ft 3 is known as 'Shorty', the biggest danger is attitude sickness. This is especially unpleasant for the referee, who is 5 ft 9.

Should the ref. also get trampled underfoot, two free shots are usually awarded.

## All-in Wrestling Injuries
Despite its seemingly high level of violence, this sport is one of the least dangerous, unless you happen to be the Chernobyl Champion,

who recently won a contest by three balls, two noses and a fall-out.

## Football Injuries
The bane of football, is of course, the 'professional foul', when, in a carefully rehearsed move, a member of the team sneaks round on the blind side of the referee and systematically nips the opposing team's testicles with an adjustable spanner. Also known as 'closing down your opponent'. Often permanently.

## The Footballer and Mental Trauma
Much has been written on the psychological aspects of belonging to a team. In such a lot of ways, belonging to any team is like belonging to a tribe or peer-group, where your companions are a cohort of like-minded people who mirror your own hopes and aspirations. And here we come to the very nub of a problem that haunts the professional footballer, for it holds the key as to whether he is to be accepted into this closest-knit of families.

Can he *gob*?

The psychological trauma which besets a man who is lacking in this, the most basic of the footballer's art, cannot be underestimated, especially if he's just cost his club £800,000.

He has watched his peers effortlessly void their windpipes with little more than a lazy flick of the tongue. And he? All he can manage is an ineffectual drool.

His decline is inevitable. Heads will turn away to denote that he is a man alone. No more splashing with the lads in the bath. A call into the manager's office. A screamed diatribe about letting down the directors. A thinly veiled threat . . . 'No gob, no job'.

He'll try anything, but his demise is assured. A few sad seasons in the lower divisions only puts off the inevitable. Finally, the day comes when he has to hang up his boots for the last time and ends up being a chartered surveyor, where the ability to gob is not yet obligatory.

## Chess Injuries
Sadly, a much more frequent occurrence nowadays. Aggressive Chess was first used by Russian Grandmasters in the early seventies. Initially, all that happened was a sly kick under the table as a variation of the opening gambit. Nothing much was done about this as it was considered part of the game. Alas, things soon worsened and led to scenes thought by many to be unworthy of

the Ancient Game. In a celebrated grudge match in Byelorussia, the defending champion, sensing perhaps that the game might be slipping away from him, bit off his opponent's nose – a move subsequently known as the Sicilian Defence. His opponent, sensing victory, later sacrificed an ear in order to get in a match-winning poke in the eye.

## 'The Fun Marathon'

'Fun Marathon'? This marriage of words is about as happy a juxtaposition as 'The Jolly Fragmentation Bomb' and I can tell you that if we find the ways of the Japanese a little strange, I had to treat an Oriental tourist for multiple cuts and bruises and also explain, in not very good Japanese, how it came about that he'd been run over by a stampede of middle-aged men dressed up as Donald Duck and Pluto. Fortunately for our country's reputation, he assumed it was the equivalent of a Japanese TV Game Show, which come to think of it, is the nearest definition I've heard.

Medical tips? Just one. Drink lots of fluid beforehand (beer, Pimms, etc). Try really hard for the first 100 yards. Then look distressed and wait for the St John's Ambulance men.

## Boxing

*Does it have long-term harmful effects?*

This one can never be proved clinically, but as one old world champion was heard to say to another:

'Spinfer jib-jab conya lefhook podder diffy wggy wof. Wasser-matter jugot braydamdge?'

To which the other, smiling in what I believe is described as a laid-back manner, replied:

'Braydamdge?? Lissen sonfabitch. Naffle woffle lefhook notcha gribbly wok twennysik millyou dollrs.'

To which, of course, there is little reply.

## Occupational Diseases

It is an unfortunate fact that some occupations themselves land themselves to a risk of disease. Everyone has heard of 'Tennis Elbow' but what about 'Car-Seller's Clutch' and 'Gardener's Mulch'?

Social medicine is uncovering more and more of these job-related diseases. Why don't you have a bit of fun and see if you've got one of these:

## Welshman's Leek

A little known infestation that affects miners in the Rhondda Coalfield. Manifesting itself as a green and white hairy swelling, it can grow to quite enormous lengths before it starts to peel.

For some reason, the Welsh, who let's face it, can be frightfully odd, take great pride in these harmless protuberances and often enter them in competitions, where tradition demands that they stand round in a circle singing 'Mefanwy', as the judges come round with the tape measure. The great secret, I am told, is to get the thing in prime condition for the show before it drops off.

## Mason's Hand Shake

It is said that one of the ways masons recognise each other in the street, is by the most invariable presence of this curious tremor. One can only hazard a guess as to its cause and although one might have one's suspicions one can't really get to the truth of the matter unless one actually gets admitted to the local lodge, which one would try but one would find very difficult, especially as one has never been proposed, but that's something one just has to accept. Anyway, who the hell wants to be a mason?

## Farmer's Beef Mountain Fever

This scourge of the last century, is making an unwelcome return to some of the remote areas of Suffolk. Caused by a mite that usually lives quietly under stones, it can, if disturbed, cause mayhem by leaping up the trouser of the unsuspecting farm-worker and with a single nip, can cause the para-sympathetic 'beef-mountain' effect. This unfortunate condition, without being too painful, can be terribly inconvenient, since the sufferer has to conduct this day to day business in a somewhat stooped manner, as well as causing absolute havoc when being measured for a suit.

## Bandleader's Bugle

In the Golden Era of Swing, it was very common to see the band-leader attempting to coax the very best out of his ensemble by indulging in a lot of leaping about and waving of arms. Why they felt constrained to do this, I don't know, but then I'm not a band-leader. What I do know is that it led to the extremities of the body becoming very oedematous, or in common parlance, squidgy. If untreated, the condition worsened, until the day would come when the band-leader would go down with the dreaded Band-leader's Bugle, so-called because whenever they sat down, they invariably emitted a loud and extremely piercing note, which, depending on the severity of the affliction, could go all the way up to F natural.

The effect when you got the whole lot of them together for dinner, for example, could be quite extraordinary. As they sat down, the unwary listener could be forgiven for thinking he'd been listening to an undisciplined version of 'Tiger Rag', which soon mutated, as they shuffled around adjusting their chairs, into a fairly random rendition of 'Don't Bring Lulu'.

Glen Miller was a notorious sufferer and legend has it that 'Chatenooga Choo-Choo' was composed quite by accident on the back of a donkey.

Sometimes, a particular social setting encourages a whole crop of occupational diseases to merge at the same time. The link is not always so obvious as to the classic 'Old Rectory Syndrome' – the triad of *Housemaid's Knee, Parson's Nose* and *Barmaid's Bottom* – which has such a pernicious effect on the ecclesiatical life of Victorian Lincolnshire until the introduction of a series of fines.

This being a book for all the family, propriety prevents me from doing anything other than just mentioning *Brewer's Yeast, Baker's Crust and Butcher's Sausage*.

## Going Abroad

Going abroad, of course, represents one of the most distasteful things one has to do in order to get warm.

In the olden days, things were somewhat easier, since contact with the natives was limited to sacking and pillage, and of course you still got your sun-tan.

The constant curse of the intrepid traveller are diarrhoea, vomiting and generalised galloping gut-rot. This is usually the result of large numbers of people being cooped up in places for long periods of time, such as Gatwick Airport.

### The Flight

Once you are safely on board the aircraft, you will notice the air hostesses position themselves at various strategic places and start to make strange signs and signals to you. On no account wave back, because this is one of their most important tasks – to let you know the position of the emergency sick-bags. You might think that this is being unnecessarily dramatic, but work out for

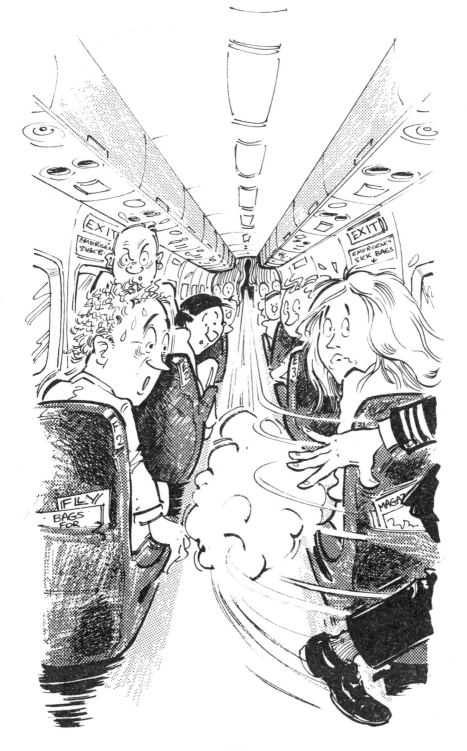

yourselves the crisis on board a non-stop flight to Agadir when you find that they've already been filled up – or, if you're travelling tourist class, that they haven't been changed from the last flight.

So the first rule of air travel must be to locate and grab a seat near the emergency sick-bags. They're usually positioned over the escape door signs.

Everyone, admit it or not, has a certain degree of disquiet when it comes to mounting those aircraft steps. In the case of one group of people, however, such feelings on boarding an aircraft amount to nothing less than sheer terror. The potential effect that an unfortunate individual of this category may have on the rest of the passengers can be well imagined, especially when he's the co-pilot.

It has to be repeated time and time again, however, that flying is statistically the safest way of travelling by air.

How to conquer this phobia? Fortunately, there are now aversion therapy courses availble for those who really want to conquer their dread of flying.

Starting off with comparatively routine flights, the danger element is gradually increased through carefully stepped increments, such as rapid depressurisation and shortage of fuel, until the advanced patient, once a mass of jelly, has so conquered his fear, that he sips a Campari during total engine failure and subsequent ditching in the Bay of Biscay.

Medically speaking, I wouldn't want to stop anyone going abroad if they're really set on it and indeed most countries do have a fully qualified nurse, but do remember to pop in to see the doctor to have your tetanus, typhus, typhoid, paratyphoid, polio, hepatitis and cholera jabs. Remember also, as you lie stretched out on some sun-drenched beach, clutching your anti-diarrhoea tablets, that the sharp little bite you felt on your exposed and semi-scorched left leg could be nothing more than the greeting of a harmless fly. Or it could be a deadly jellyfish or leg-eating spider. These, of course, are very rare . . . as are snakes, leeches, scorpions, amoebic dysentery, leprosy, lassa fever and lost luggage.

Again, without generalising too much, it's best to give some areas a total miss. I've heard bad reports of the following:

'Meet the Ton Ton Macout' Holiday & Leisure Tours of Haiti.
'Meet the Locals' tours, arranged by the New York Subway Dept.
Kalahari Surfboard Holidays.
Real Ale Pub Crawls in Saudi Arabia.

# Sweltering Parts

## A Catalogue of Tropical Diseases

If you're still intent on travelling further south than the Dover Ferry, I feel it's only fair to point out that although we have to put up with cold noses and hot flushes, they are relatively quite lovely compared with some of the nasties awaiting your arrival in foreign parts, often announcing themselves as you are still descending the aircraft steps.

*Delhi Belly* needs no introduction, whereas its lesser known brother, *Bombay Dick*, perhaps does, although it is wont to make its own introduction before you've reached passport control. *Brazzaville Bottom* sadly needs no introduction whatsoever and can be hell to keep the flies off, while *Dahomey Drip* and *Rift Valley Rot* are two ugly sisters you would certainly not wish to take to the ball, particularly as that's where it can cause the most trouble anyway.

*Fiji Squeejy* can make your life hell and must be allowed to dry out, while sufferers are prevented from returning to the Mother Country by quarantine laws and in any case, requires many months' immersion in turps for a sure cure.

*Wombooka's Verruca* can spread like the clappers via infected visa application forms and if victims of this terrible scourge even manage to get back to the UK they sadly have to be put down because of EEC regulations.

*Congo Dongo* can remain a permanent souvenir of embassy cocktail parties and can be a serious impediment to career advancement in the Diplomatic Corps; and it goes without saying that the object horror of *Umbonga's Disease* should preclude any intrepid traveller from sharing a sleeping-bag with anyone who's had any contact whatsoever with Umbonga.

You'd have to travel a long way (and fortunately, you generally do) in order to meet anything as nasty as *Ganges Tongue*, which, together with *Gambian Gum*, will give your dentist a fairly torrid time.

I do hope this little pot-pourri hasn't put you off too much from donning your khakis. It's only fair to add that in a normal fortnight, you'd probably avoid at least one or two of the above, as long as you took some basic precautions, such as not leaving the hotel or drinking anything.

# The Bit You've Been Waiting For: Sexual Medicine

# Your Sexual Problems Answered

Bringing your sexual problems into the surgery represents one of doctor's greatest challenges. He will listen to descriptions of your most intimate and sometimes frankly embarrassing moments. It is vital that you should be able to be straightforward and honest about your problems, because although you may think you're grossly inadequate, doctor is there to help and in any case is used to dealing with grossly inadequate people.

It would be wrong of me if I said that all my medical colleagues were equally trained or indeed suited to help you with sexual matters. Try to gauge for yourself whether he is 'on the ball', so to speak. Some quite subtle powers of observation are often needed. Let me explain. As you attempt to unburden yourself of your 'problem', you might see doctor taking notes. This is a good sign. If he is making drawings, this is a bad sign. If he gets *you* to do the drawings, make your excuses and leave. Another example. Is he nodding encouragingly? Good. Is he nodding encouragingly and over-salivating? *Not* good.

Sexual problems are multifarious and difficult to put into neat compartments. But after some years of study, I feel they fall into the following categories:

*a* His fault.
*b* Her fault.
*c* Mother's fault.

This last category falls beyond the scope of this modest volume. It includes strange things like the Oedipus Complex, so-called after the block of flats in Athens where it was first discovered. As far as I'm concerned, it's a Greek problem and they can clear up their own mess.

## A) His fault
*i* Premature arrival.
This shortcoming can arise from a deep-seated fear of being late. Most experts agree that the solution to this vexed and common problem is to start earlier.

*ii* Late arrival.
Apart from being a worry, this can be extremely boresome, especially if you've got better things to do. Late arrival usually

arises if you've missed your connection. Check your partner's timetable, so you can both be in bed at the same time.

*iii* Non-arrival.
The most annoying of this annoying trio, although it can give the female partner a bit of time to catch up on some reading, doing the ironing, etc. For the male, however, it is a real worry. Often caused by signal failure further up the line. Have a specialist check your rolling stock.

*iv* Failure to maintain an eruption.
Very upsetting and can involve a great deal of hanging about. Its most common cause is realisation by the male partner that he is missing the Cricket Highlights. This is really an occasion to seek psycho-sexual advice from an expert like Richie Benaud.

*v* Failure to remove socks.
This should be self-explanatory. However, it has to be said that the wearing of socks does not in itself prevent full interaction taking place and indeed can be useful in gaining extra anchorage. Having said that, best to take them off and argue about it afterwards.

*vi* 'I'm sure it's me, doctor'.
One of the male partner's greatest fears is that the failure of a physical relationship is sometimes his fault. This is, of course, one of those gross over-simplifications. It is *always* his fault.

For the alert male, therefore, here are a few bad signs to look out for:

– Yawning or polishing nails during foreplay.
– You notice there's another man in the bed.
– You notice there are two other men in the bed.
– While you're thrashing about, she announces she's emigrating.
– Erogenous zones become Total Exclusion Zones.
– She says, 'That was sensational, Harry!' This is great news for Harry. Your name is Edward.

## B) Her fault
No it's not. It's your fault.

# Some Sexual Terms and Expressions Explained

## The Missionary Position

As every schoolboy knows, when Charles Livingstone was sent out to Africa, he was absolutely hell-bent on spreading Christianity.

In 1874, however, while having a go at the Wombonga Tribe, he fell madly in love with a man called Stanley. (Nobody knows his surname.)

All went well until some Wombongan Elders decided to surprise them with some early-morning coconut. They were deeply shocked at the sight that befell them. This was the Missionary Position.

To this very day, the only words of English these primitive people speak are, 'This is another fine mess you've got me into, Stanley.'

Not surprisingly, the whole experience put them off both sex and Christianity.

## Sexual Four-Ply

An Australian contraption made out of wood, whose use I don't feel we need go into.

## Casual Sex

In the days when things were awfully chic, casual sex was all the rage. During the middle of it all, for example, it was quite common for one of the partners to pop out to take the dog for a walk.

Casual sex died a natural death when things got so chic that both partners would decide to take the dog out for a walk.

## Aural Sex

This is the sensual gratification gained from using one or both ears. It generally starts off as a gentle bit of lobe-sucking, but very quickly gets out of control and is characterised by grunts and screams as bits of the ear get chewed off.

It has now largely gone out of fashion, which is a shame, for apart from being one of life's little pleasures, it represented a most efficient way of keeping your ears clean and free of wax.

## The Point of No Return

During sexual congress, a point is eventually reached after which it would be imprudent to get up and make the coffee.

Experienced exponents in the art of love-making can postpone the onset of this magical slalom almost indefinitely. Unfortunately, the less experienced male, either due to anxiety or worry, gets there sooner than he'd ideally like, usually while toppling over trying to pull his shoes off.

It is often a useful tip for the floundering tyro who's prone to premature explosions, to conjure up certain images so that he may keep things going a little longer. Here are some suggestions that have a proven track record.

**1.** A plate of cold semolina, complete with dollop of jam.

**2.** Benito Mussolini.

**3.** A hippopotamus on the job.

## Yo-Ho-Ho : A Brief History of Marine Sex

This curious and little-known corner of the sexual landscape gained a huge popularity following the success of E.M. Forster's stirring tales of Captain Fellatio Hornblower.

Separated from their wives for months and years on end, the indomitable captain instituted certain disciplines which ensured that his men beat the French and also made lifelong friendships.

## Noises in the Night

If there's one thing that separates man from woman, it's the noises they make during intercourse.

Women will give vent to their feelings by seemingly answering an unheard question. Hence, she will often be heard to exclaim 'Oh yes' or 'Oh no', sometimes, 'Oh my God' and on occasions, 'Have you finished, you great Wally?'

Men, on the other hand, tend to be less florid in their pronouncements and limit themselves to facial expressions of grim determination, not unlike one who is profoundly constipated, interspersed with occasional imprecations such as 'Herrgh . . . Herrgh . . . Oogh-oogh – aaar . . . Hoo-Hoo-Hoo – aaaaargh . . . .' In fact, much the same sound as an orang-utang might make whilst indulging in a similar pursuit.

It needs only to be added that women sometimes sound as if they're going to die of ecstasy and men always sound as if they're going to die of a heart attack.

# A Quick Whip-through Sexual Perversions

## Fetishist

A fetish may be defined as the regarding of something with an irrational reverence. Thus, some people might have a foot fetish, others a frog fetish and yet others may just be misguided young Conservatives.

The point is that no fetish is wrong; indeed, there are probably as many of them as there are young Conservatives.

Here are a couple of lesser known ones:

*a* Sexo-Horticultural

Typically a middle-aged man, often a VAT Inspector and seemingly leading a normal and healthy life, but in his secret hours he knows he is irresistibly drawn to and has an unnatural interest in flora with large pods.

You will sometimes see this sad figure, who we know as a Podophile, wandering around the Kew Garden Hot House, seemingly at random; but a closer look will reveal that the orchids and bromeliads hold no interest for him, because he only has eyes for one thing. *Porchyphylla enorma*, a member of the Banana family, which I can tell you has extremely large pods.

With careful counselling, podophiles can be gently weaned off their obsession by way of hollyhocks and snapdragons, and in a surprisingly short time can walk through a garden centre without getting arrested.

*b* Fossil Worship

A similar group of people, usually worried about their virility, who can hardly walk around the British Museum's Paleolithic exhibit and leave without some sort of bone in their pocket.

## Sado-Masochism and Bondage

Sado-masochism is another way of never having to say you're sorry. It is often associated with a strange desire of wanting to be tied up, generally in a special place called The House of Bondage – something first experienced by the Israelites during their days in ancient Egypt. Moses, who by all accounts was a bit of an old stick about these things, decided enough was enough and took the lot of them to cool off in the desert for forty years. This therapy is somewhat impractical nowadays, although a good idea is to get out and meet a few people. How about the Young Conservatives?

## Flagellation

This gained much notoriety after the advent of the infamous 'Wheals of Fire', a tale of undergrads who got into training for the 1924 Olympics by whipping themselves into a frenzy around the quad at Lady Mary College, Oxford.

Their methods, although considered controversial at the time, were vindicated when they not only came away with the medals, but went on to become senior government ministers and distinguished Soviet spies.

## Group Sex

Group sex is not strictly a perversion, but because it is so rampant in places such as Hendon, I feel it deserves at least a mention.

As with so many of the unwholesome aspects of contemporary society, group sex owes its origins to the permissive sixties, although how people of that age maintain their enthusiasm is a mystery.

The ritual at these sessions follows a fairly set pattern. Everyone generally gathers around the kitchen table, drinking tea and having a general chin-wag, until someone surreptitiously slips out his dentures and lays them on the table. This is the signal the others have been waiting for.

Within seconds, the table is covered with discarded dentures, hearing aids, toupees, glass eyes and false noses. Having thus made their intentions clear, they adjourn to the drawing-room for more athletic pursuits, generally leaving one of their number, who hasn't really grasped what's going on, to put on the kettle.

The mayhem in the drawing-room can go on for some time, but things are generally brought to a halt in time for the Afternoon Play or the Omnibus Edition of The Archers.

## Pulling the Mangabey

Let's face it, pulling the Mangabey has been with us ever since Man discovered he had one. Let me assure you, however, that there is absolutely no scientific evidence to suggest that pulling the Mangabey can lead to any long-lasting physical damage, except, of course, going blind.

Most males are aware of their Mangabeys from an early age, but it is not until their early teens that the dirty boy in the class demonstrates that it can be pulled. This is quite normal and even desirable, as it stops him wanting to play horrible games.

However, dangers do lurk ahead.

Whereas Mangabey pulling can be a great comfort to the growing boy, problems begin to occur when the pimply youth has grown into a full man and, to put it bluntly, instead of pulling the birds, he's still pulling his Mangabey.

Its full horror is manifested in married life. You see, what a lot of men don't realise is that women don't *have* a Mangabey. Why, I don't know, but there you are. That is not to say that they wouldn't *like* to have one. And this is where the problem lies. Mangabey Envy.

If you want a simple answer, I'm afraid there isn't one. Mangabey counselling can sometimes help, but I fear that the problem is too deeply seated for simple solutions.

What a woman would want with a Mangabey, I don't know. My feeling is that the only thing you can do is gently to explain to her that it's yours and she's not having it.

# Contraception

## The Cap
Sometimes worn on the head by the male to remind him no precautions are being used by the female. A sexual equivalent of the knotted handkerchief, which, by the way, is useless as a contraceptive.

In order to make doubly sure that neither partner forgets, the cap is sometimes worn by both male and female. This is known as 'Going Dutch'.

## The Safe Period
This is an indeterminate length of time, during which neither partner is interested in sex.

*Advantages*
a No one gets blamed if it doesn't work.
b No mess.

## Spermicidal Jelly
One of the more modern forms of contraception. However, it must never be considered as the main line of defence and must always be used in conjunction with other forms of contraception such as the French Lettuce.

*Advantages*
*a* Like all jellies, can be kept in the fridge.
*b* Goes very well with ice-cream

## The Rhythm Method
In the days before modern technology brought us such things as jellies and ice-cream, people had to rely on what became known as the Rhythm Method, so-called because the couple timed their endeavours to something like a Strauss waltz, which is why this method subsequently became known as the Congress of Vienna. 'The Blue Danube' was a great favourite. Its theme might have been written for the part: 'Da-*da*-da-da-*da* . . . Boop Boop, Boop Boop, etc.'

*Advantages*
   a) Soothing and aesthetically pleasing.
   b) You don't have to run down to the chemist.

*Disadvantages*
*a* Not absolutely safe because of:
   **1** Record getting stuck.
   **2** Record accidentally being put on at 78 rpm.
   **3** Ill-judged choice of music, such as 'The William Tell Overture' or 'Minute Waltz'.
*b* Some people decide to splash out and hire a chamber orchestra. Although this often starts out as a good idea, its presence can become intrusive, especially if the room isn't terribly suited, such as a bed-sit.

## The Condom
The condom is the most ancient form of contraception known to man and happily has now truly come out of the closet. For too long they were considered to be unmentionables, only obtainable at back-street barbers and sleazy chemists.

But thanks to TV chat shows, they have now become the motif of the eighties – a favourite topic for discussion at dinner parties and now obtainable at any reputable florist's or delicatessen.

Their main drawback is that they still look so awful – great big pink things with a wart on the end. One tends to think that things haven't improved since the olden days when condoms were made out of pigs' bladders. This didn't go down too well with Jewish people and wasn't too popular with the pigs either.

# Should I Have a Sperm Count?

At first glance, having your sperm counted would seem a strange thing to want to do. But just as some people worry about their weight, others like to keep a finger on their sperm. Apart from all that, it's quite a good thing to do for that rainy afternoon.

Before we go any further, perhaps we ought to explain things a little with some basic physiology.

So what is a sperm?

Well, without being too scientific, a sperm, or to give it its full scientific name, the spermoplod, is a squiggly little thing that looks a bit like a tadpole, although the two should never be confused. If you're not sure which is which, keep a mixture in a jar of water on the window-sill. The ones that grow into frogs aren't sperm.

In a lighter vein, I might add that in the dark days of medicine, it used to be thought that this tadpole swam up the female's floppy tubes, ate the egg and grew into a frog. This has now been largely discounted.

We now know that the quickest swimmer among these nippy little beggars whizzes up the floppy tube until it finds the omelette or egg, wiggles its way in and – Hey Presto! – the long process that could end up with a place at Winchester begins.

Back to our sperm count. In some males, the number of viable spermoplods is unusually low. For many years this remained a mystery. But modern techniques in electron microscopy have shown a most unlikely culprit – the Bladder Beetle. This voracious creature stalks its unsuspecting prey by remaining motionless in the darker recesses of the urino-genital tract and when it spots its victim – a sperm which has become detached from the herd, or maybe a wounded straggler – leaps out and gobbles it up before legging it back to the bladder.

## Donating the Sperm

Because of lack of resources within the NHS, the giving of a sperm sample often takes place in the same room as is used by the blood donors.

Always let the nurse know which one you've come for. There is nothing more off-putting for the sperm-donor than to see nurse bearing down on him with a tourniquet. Conversely, donating your blood is quite horrid enough without having to provide a sperm sample at the same time.

The actual mechanics of sperm donation can, of course, be

embarrassing. But try to remember that the other twenty or so people lined up with you are trying to do exactly the same thing as you are. Just look straight ahead and concentrate on the matter in hand. Most establishments try to provide inspiration with a few well-chosen murals of great figures from the past, such as Thomas Cranmer.

## Counting the Sperm: the Difficult Bit

If you bump into someone at a cocktail party and sense there is something in his eyes – a faraway and oracular look – that tells you that here is someone rather special, the chances are you're talking to a sperm-counter, or, as they prefer to be called, Sperm Totalling Operative.

A breed apart, they tend to keep to themselves, preferring their own company and quietly talking shop in their own private language.

What makes these people so special?

Imagine being slumped over a high-resolution magnifying glass, sometimes for days on end, totting up unnumbered squigglies. It almost defies belief, doesn't it? No computer or fancy adding machines for *them*. For it is a tradition among sperm totalling operatives that they can use only the naked eye and the fingers of the right hand for their demanding task.

Of course, if it were just a matter of counting up to 40-50 million sperm, then anybody could do it. What people forget is that those 40-50 million sperm are all swimming around like demented Duncan Goodhews, for it is a scientific fact that sperm don't like to be disturbed.

So imagine, those of you out there who want to join the freemasonry of the Sperm Totallers, that you are in the middle of a count and have reached, say, 38,476,404. You see something move out of the corner of your eye. Is it a rogue sperm that's wandered off on its own, or just a bit of banana? Have I counted it? You start to panic, because without wishing to be offensive, all sperm, let alone bits of banana, tend to look exactly the same. By the time you've sorted this lot out, the other 38,476,404 have whizzed off somewhere else and you end up having to start again.

It's no wonder, therefore, that Sperm Totallers are only allowed to work for a maximum of seven consecutive days, after which they are grounded and must spend a compulsory period for rest and recreation at Sperm House, just outside Glastonbury.

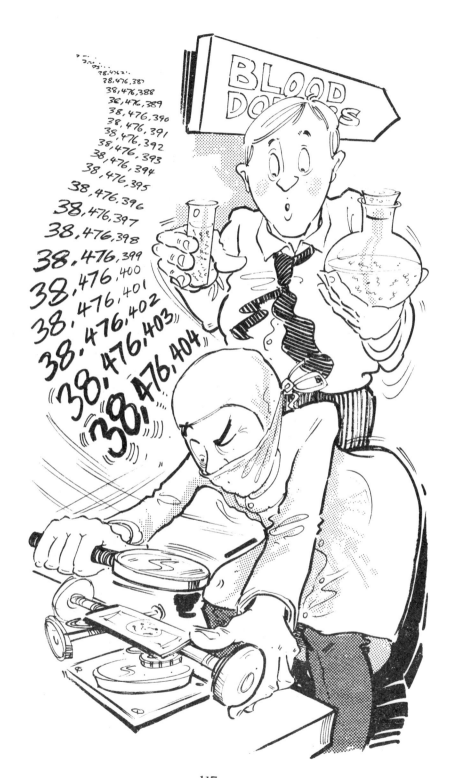

117

# Going Into Hospital

Hospitals, let's face it, can be pretty daunting places. But an enforced stay there needn't necessarily be unpleasant, as long as one realises that, for most of us, it is the nearest one gets to doing time in prison.

You arrive there, clutching your pitiful bundle of possessions, sign on the dotted and are marched off to your cell-block.

To make you feel at home, your new abode is given a name that has a reassuring and homely ring to it, such as C6 or Bromide Ward.

In any event, to keep your morale up, you are then generally stripped and given a number which you wear round your wrist. On no account lose this, for it could mean the difference between having your haemorrhoids done, which you came in for, and having your kidneys whipped, which you didn't and moreover, could ruin your stay.

Well now, the formalities are over and they have finally left you alone. So there you are, propped up in your bed, feeling perfectly healthy and wondering why you have begun to sob.

Get to know the rest of the inmates in your cell-block. They will have a variety of ailments, from gall-stones, through back-ache, to thinking they're turning into a giant squid. Make sure, if possible, that your bed is as far away as possible from the man who thinks he's turning into a giant squid.

As you glance around, you will notice that some patients have lots of tubes stuck into them. These need not concern you and are merely there to remind doctors which patients have already had their operations.

Sooner or later, a hush will descend upon the place, This signifies the arrival of the consultoid. He is a very, very clever and wise man and for this reason he often wears half-moon spectacles and a non-matching bow-tie.

Running along in his wake and in strict pecking order, are his senior registrar and houseboy. Each are hanging on his every word, for one day, they too will become consultoids.

To avoid the embarrassment of having to talk to you, consultoids will generally behave as if they are deaf and dumb. Hence, he will approach your bed, smile benignly, then turn to no one in particular and say something like 'Which one is this?' As the houseboy gives him a detailed history of your case, he will stand over you and, in a messianic way, close his eyes as if trying to make contact with the Hereafter and poke about with the affected part of your body. Bearing in mind that there may be six pairs of eyes on you, how should you react? Never show discomfort, rather, turn your head aside peer into the middle distance and let a contented smile play upon your lips, as if recalling the pleasure of seeing an old friend once again – not the easiest thing, especially if you've come in to have your piles done.

Your time in hospital can be generally divided into three time zones.

1 Feeling great.

2 Doctors making you better.

3 Recovering from doctors making you feel better.

## Feeling Great

Feeling great whilst in hospital can last for varying amounts of time, but generally speaking, it has a directly inverse relationship with how efficient the place is. Putting it another way, the more inefficient the hospital, the longer you'll be left alone, or even better, forgotten about, and the longer you'll feel great. Judicious journeys to the lavvy, timed to coincide with the arrival of anyone in a white coat, can keep this going for days, if not weeks. Make the most of this period, because sooner or later, they'll catch up with you and start 'making you better'.

## Making you better

This involves making you feel extremely ill, thus giving you justification for being in hospital. It is often associated with a roaring temperature, violent headache, mixed in with prolonged bouts of vomiting.

You will often have confirmation of how much better you are when you hear a man in a while coat saying, 'We're very pleased with you!' or, 'He's looking a little brighter today'. You smile weakly, aware that your face must be resembling a traffic light, alternating between red and green, depending on whether it is registering your tropical temperature or the imminent return of monsoonal vomiting. The lights turn to 'go', and with as much dignity as you can muster, you turn your head to one side and fill up the bowl again. With *what*, you don't know, since all you've managed to eat since they've started making you feel better is two segments of orange and a fig. For some reason, this manifestation of what you believe is the act of snuffing it, produces a reaction of profound satisfaction from the man in the white coat. Nodding with vigorous approbation, he'll exclaim something like 'Jolly good!' or 'Well done!', as if the reappearance of two segments of orange and the remains of a fig is all the confirmation he needs that all's going to plan.

The traffic light, for no obvious reason, tires of being green and returns to a comfortable vermillion and you actually find yourself trying to apologize for the exhibition you've just laid on, except that the word that emerges resembles, 'Thurgoo', since your tongue has got stuck to your palate.

## Recovery from Being Treated

Your road to recovery can be a long and arduous one. Its length depends on your will to get out in one piece and indeed, whether they decide you're not quite better and need a little more treatment, which can set back your recovery considerably.

Perhaps the first sign that your body – like a dandelion run over by a steam-roller, but still be determined to flower – is returning to normal, can be a strange sensation which you eventually trace to your nostrils, which are trying to close of their own accord. After a few more seconds, a cause suggests itself – an odd smell that starts to prevade the consciousness, awakening feelings of primordial fear. The metallic rattle echoing along the ward is like the tolling of a death knell. The dinner trolley is here.

You try and make yourself as invisible as you can, slithering down into the sheets like a pyjama'd chameleon. The rattle comes closer and stops by your bed. You have stopped breathing and in a flash realise what it must be to live in a totalitarian state. Suddenly, the air is desecrated by an accent that can only be produced when a lady from the Phillipines comes to this country and decides to settle in Birmingham.

There have, of course, been countless jokes made at the expense of hospital food, but they are all built on a great misconception. The fact is that hospital food is not something to eat, but something to *do*.

You see, in many ways, being in hospital is like being subjected to a never-ending plane journey. You have to sit there, taking your medicine and wait for the time you can get off. But until that moment arrives, you are unutterably, indisputably, unbearingly, inconsolably and irreversibly BORED.

So nibble at your lunch, fight off the nausea and keep telling yourself that it is occupying several minutes of your day and anything, *anything* is better than strapping on the headphones again, knowing that the only thing you can get is Radio Two.

This boredom drives people to do strange things. Take a look around you and you'll see great hunks of machismo, complete with gold medallions disappearing into chestfuls of designer hair, devouring back-numbers of 'The Fuchsia Society Bulletin', not to mention fragile old grannies, complete with voluminous shawl, getting stuck into 'Secrets of the Scrum'.

And so, slowly, you begin to feel like your old self. It is around this time that you begin to detest your visitors.

Visiting someone in hospital is, of course, a meaningless ritual, since in general terms, both parties wish they were somewhere else. So how to deal with these unwanted guests?

As they arrive, a good ruse is to feign a relapse. This is what to do:

Close your eyes, get a good mouthful of dribble going and as they reach your bed, let your head loll around a bit and release your dribble at a steady rate so that it slurps gently out of the corner of your mouth to form a pool in the hollow just beneath your Adam's Apple. Then open your eyes as widely as they can go and say, 'My God, I'm late for an appointment!' Then close your eyes again and recommence dribbling.

If done convincingly, your visitors will generally study their shoelaces, before agreeing that perhaps they might go for a curry.

So finally, the magical day arrives when it's time for you to go – with a song in your heart and possibly minus a kidney. You go round saying your goodbye, realising quite suddenly, that you know someone by their first names.

There's Sid, who you've just spend three weeks lying next to – Sid, loved by everybody – the original Salt of the Earth, with his homespun philosophy, native good sense and unfailing good humour and who hated enough to kill.

And not just the patients. There's old Lenny, the morgue attendant, always whistling 'The Happy Wanderer' and liking nothing more than to share a joke. You hated *him* as well. As these thoughts are tumbling through your mind as you approach the front exit of the hospital.

You're still thinking of them all as your nose smashes against the door that, when you entered the hospital, opened automatically.

You regain consciousness. You are lying in a bed. A voice impinges into your consciousness, summoning you to lunch.

# Your Very Own Operation

One of the less attractive prospects of your stay in hospital is that somewhere down the line, a complete stranger is going to forcibly render you unconscious, after which, someone else is going to hack a way through your body wall and tear, scratch, strip, slice, snip, skin, rip, slash, slit and sever his way through what was once your own sole property.

Try not to let this prey on your mind.

You will almost invariably find that your operation will be timed for 10.30 in the morning. This is because surgeons like to have coffee and a fag before starting on anything too energetic or indeed, messy. This still gives them plenty of time before they want to knock off for lunch. Surgeons will generally make every effort to get you finished before they get peckish, although if you're not quite done before lunch, they nearly always leave someone behind just to keep an eye on things, like a porter, while they wander off to the canteen.

Now, back to *you*. Anyone who has had an operation will know that you won't be allowed breakfast or supper the night before. This is because the hospital might quite reasonably feel that if you don't make it through the op., the cost of those two meals would constitute a rather unnecessary waste of government money.

As the morning progresses, the nursing staff will be very supportive by saying that 'there's absolutely nothing to worry about' every two or three minutes. Further solace can be gained by them whispering to each other, 'He was such a nice man', as they tidy up your belongings.

Relief will finally come to you in the shape of the *Pre-Med*. A quick jab in the buttocks and your world will be soon transformed. A deep calmness will start to enfold you. Never again will you feel such a sense of inner peace as you lie there, bombed out of your skull. This is where the giggles set in and reach a crescendo as you are put on a trolley and let off down the corridor, serene now in the knowledge that you could face a firing squad and still launch into 'The Sun Has Got His Hat On', if only you could stop screeching with laughter.

Whilst in this state, it is only fair to point out that you may well start to babble, cry, swear or fart – often simultaneously. This is frequently taped by the theatre staff, although you may be sure that it is done in the strictest confidentiality and is only rarely played back over the hospital radio to entertain the other patients.

Usually, the last thing you remember before submitting your virgin pink flesh to the knife, is the anaesthetist advancing towards you and saying, 'There's absolutely nothing to worry about'. You might just hear the surgeon mutter, 'Has anyone seen my specs?' before you giggle yourself into oblivion.

The next thing you are aware of is a throbbing pain and a tube stuck up your nose. This tells you you've had your operation. You try to focus your eyes in order to check whether you've pulled through. You find you are alone with your pain and your tube. You try to call for a nurse, but all you can manage is a longish nose-bubble, which not only won't go away, but also goes in and out in time with your pitiful sobs.

You are on the road to recovery.

## How to Treat Your Dentist

Teeth are amongst the most clever of all the bits of the body. Just imagine what it would be like if they hadn't been invented.

Meryl Streep would look extremely silly for a start. And imagine sitting down to that romantic candle-lit dinner, lisping sweet nothings to each other before having to psyche yourself up to tackle a T-bone steak.

Or back at your place and that shy first kiss ruined by a chunk of lobster en Crut that's defeated the attentions of your over-worked gums.

Most important of all, the invention of teeth has given useful employment to a group of people who otherwise would find it difficult to hold down a job – your dentist.

Somehow, dentists have always had to reputation of being out and out sadists, whose idea of a pleasant day's toil is to inflict untold misery on their charges, before going home to bite the canary's head off. This is patently untrue, especially as most dentists don't even keep pet brids.

Dentists are often asked how on earth they can look down peoples' mouths all day. The sensitive dentist would answer that he is more concerned with the fact that he spends his day with total strangers looking up his nose. You see, dentists are professionals and are chronically worried about the state of their nose-holes. You probably don't realise it, but the reason he asks you to rinse out so often, is so that he can grab one of those funny looking mirrors to take a quick peek to make sure that there is nothing nasty hanging out of his left nostril.

What you don't realise, of course, is that the one thing the dentist wants above all, is to be loved. He knows, for example, that you don't really want to come and see him. He knows that *nobody* really wants to come and see him. He tries to make things easier for you with tapes of Neil Diamond and Richard Kleiderman, but nothing can change the unalterable fact that, all things considered, you'd prefer to be in bed with mumps.

In order words, a dentist at work is usually close to tears. So here are a few tips to show him you care:

1 Make sure you arrive with clean teeth and arm-pits.

2 Try not to lower his spirits with depressing news. Dance gaily into his surgery, giggle skittishly and announce you've been up all night with toothache.

3 Pretend you like Neil Diamond and Richard Kleiderman.

4 Tell him you think dentists are grossly underpaid.

5 As he impales the affected tooth with his probe, try not to leap out of the chair screaming obscenities; Rather, congratulate him along the lines of, 'My word, Mr. Jenkins, I'd never have thought it was *that* one'.

6 Try not to vomit as nurse sticks the sucker down your throat. It's generally because she's attempting to change the Neil Diamond tape with her spare hand.

7 Do not, if at all possible, have stringy saliva. Dentists tend to take this as a personal affront and makes them very bad-tempered.

8 Some people have thin tongues. Some people have fat ones. But the tongues that really annoy the dentist are the ones that follow him everywhere. Imagine it. He is quietly getting on with sorting out a crater that used to be the second molar, miles away from where the tongue lives, when for now apparent reason, it slithers upwards and nestles itself warm and wetly against the dentist's little pinkie. And no matter what he does, there it is, like an amorous slug, sliming its affections over the fingers of someone who doesn't even remember your name.

9 Never bite the hand that treats you.

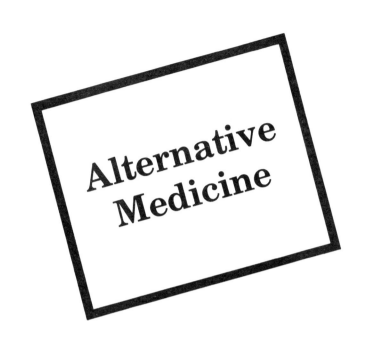

Alternative Medicine

# The Changing Pattern of Illness

Not so long ago, illness, like life itself, was less confusing than today. Short periods of malady were one's mere entitlement for weeks of slogging away at the office helping to maintain the nose-diving economy of the country. When you were ill, you were permitted a few days of well-deserved respite to feel totally sorry for yourself and to demand the complete indulgence of one's kin. You sloped languidly off to bed with a hot water bottle and dug in to wait for the doctor to arrive with a bottle of placebo.

For a few days, you'd be allowed to rule the house from your sickbed, disrupting everybody else's routine with piteous cries for fresh hot water bottles, change of sheets or squads of relations to come and clean up sick just as they were settling down for a well-earned meal. They were duty bound to sit patiently disguising their irritation and disgust while you contrarily paddled your spoon in the bread and milk before spilling it all over the pillow.

Having eventually become bored by being bedridden, skilled sufferers could usually push their luck with a period of convalescence. Sitting around in pyjamas looking waxy could be spun out to a week or so, during which time you could still demand that your food be cut up and the television moved into the room of your choice.

Convalescence usually ended when:

**1** Credibility ran out – e.g. being caught in the kitchen in the dead of night, eating your way through a bunch of bananas.
**2** District nurse arrived to give you an enema.
**3** Your announcement that you were 'still feeling a bit weak' led to your next of kin hanging herself from the banister.

Nowadays, however, much of the fun has been taken out of minor illness by the abandonment of the 'pleasure principle' – i.e. lying back in the sheets quaffing syrup of neurophosphates and listening to Desert Island Discs. The whole thing has been undermined by science which demands investigations, diagnosis and proper treatment.

As a result, a quite promising bout of biliousness is likely to be anything but relaxing. Instead of slothing around in bed devouring milk puddings, you are likely to be frogmarched up to an impersonal outpatient clinic and made to swallow four feet of rubberised cable with a light bulb on the end. Following this ordeal, you may be required to suffer a gallon of freezing cold barium being propelled vigorously up the entrails by several ladies wearing lead clothing. If there is great excitement and half the hospital come to peer at the X-ray screen, you will know they've located the light bulb.

The development of powerful modern drugs has brought several disadvantages:

*a* They may make you better horribly quickly, leaving you feeling cheated and bitter.

*b* They may send you bonkers.

*c* They may cause unsightly rashes. You may be banished from the bedroom and forced to huddle into bed with the au pair.

*d* Impotence and torrential diarrhoea may then be a problem.

Proper drugs tend to have inconvenient side-effects like wiping out all the cells in your bone marrow. Furthermore, as everyone knows, you may get hooked and need to mortgage your house and business to furnish an insatiable craving for black-market bowel regulators.

## The Holistic Alternative

Not surprisingly, many intelligent people have had their fill of orthodox medical practices, which, as they rightly point out, have caused untold suffering, denuded the world of tropical rainforests and tilted the Earth's axis, altering its climate. General practitioners and drug companies are, of course, largely to blame. Revolted by this interference in the world's ecosystem, patients are increasingly rejecting the doctor's materialist 'cause and effect' interpretation of Nature, abandoning high-tech drugs and treatment and returning to time-honoured, natural remedies like rubbing bums together in a basin of Perrier water. Weary of doctors' obsession with treating the symptom, the devotees of Alternative Medicine seek a broader, 'holistic' approach to the individual.

### What is 'Holistic'?
A holistic approach to medicine implies treating the whole person – mind, body and spirit – rather than just concentrating on the bit that's throbbing. According to this philosophy, one's being is an energy system, inseparable from the timeless, limitless energies of the cosmos, with which it should be in perfect harmony – much as it is when we take tranquillisers. Holism is a philosophy not just of medicine but of life itself.

# How Holistic Are You?

**1** Tick the things you like doing
    – making wholemeal bread;
weaving patchwork quilts;
reading about goat husbandry;
hunting pandas.

**2** Which of these are good for head-colds?
    – mustard and garlic baths;
anabolic steroids;
marijuana;
nut rissole;
ECT.

**3** Which of the following are *not* Druid shrines?
    – the Malmesbury Ring;
Lords;
Stonehenge;
Porton Down;
Bagshot.

**4** Suitable names for male children
    – Prahindra;
Mahesh Yogi;
Bertie.

**5** Which of the following is used in meditation?
    – a mantra;
a Fiat Uno;
a black mamba.

**6** Tick your favourite foods
    – lentil en croute;
hot spicy lentil;
lentil with coriander;
savoury whalebone.

**7** Which of the following are most useful in bringing about worldwide nuclear disarmament?
    – Vitamin B6;
Breast-pumps;
Ginseng;
Crocodile skin handbags;
Condoms.

It may come as something of a surprise to my loyal patients to learn that I am by no means a complete killjoy when it comes to the holistic, bone-through-the-nose approach to healing.

Indeed, I submit that it can offer distinct advantages, many of them quite lucrative.

Setting aside my slight scepticism, I now offer you a brief account of a few of the less loathsome practices available in so-called Alternative Medicine, sparing you the unnecessary offence of having to read about its more obscene disciplines (I refer particularly to 'Excreta Therapy', 'Primal Climax Treatment' and 'Zududu Beads').

# Incense and Rumbumiratnas

## Meditation
This is an ancient discipline practiced for centuries by Eastern mystics in order to find Oneness with the Universe.

Experienced meditators can achieve extraordinary feats of physiology such as slowing the heartbeat, revolving the eyeballs and making the blood pump backwards.

## Transcendental Meditation
This soothes away the stresses of everyday life – it's a must for the tense, frenetic businessman struggling to keep the order books full, the accounts balanced. Just twenty minutes' calm twice a day – not just for you but for the whole workforce. For forty minutes the factory goes still and quiet; no clattering conveyor belts, no grinding turbines, no typing. Complete calm descends. The shop steward sits under a tree swaying gently to his mantra. For the equivalent of a mere thirty-three working days each year, nobody lifts so much as a crowbar. Nobody shouts, nobody throws a wobbly and nobody gets wound up until the receiver moves in at the end of the financial year.

## Learning to Meditate
You will need:
1 Joss sticks.
2 Mantra.
3 Three hundred pounds.

## What is a Mantra?
A 'mantra' is something given to you by a Guru or specially trained psychiatric nurse. It is a word or thought upon which you let your mind settle like a butterfly – e.g. 'Rumbumiratna', 'Sausages' or 'Mugabe'.

In times of great commotion, your mantra will enable you to transcend the unruly storm and find the Inner Peace of the Unified Field. Perhaps the kids are screaming, the toilet has sprung a leak and your wife is wrestling with a man from the finance company while he struggles to untack the carpets. At such a time, retire quietly to your room, close your eyes and let the mantra lead you to the Inner Tranquillity. In some other plane of consciousness you may dimly hear the door splintering under the axe and the arrival of the police and the dogs. A great sublime calm has come upon you. This is called transcending. A warm sensation gathers on your breastbone and is spreading slowly to your navel. This is called dribbling. Far from the raging battle you perceive serenity . . . darkly, through a glass. Beyond it – the dim outline of a social worker.

## Feeling the Hara

The 'hara' lies on the body somewhere below the navel. It is our Centre of Gravity and the source of many Vital Energies. Many people like to feel the hara during meditation. Aesthetes are continually feeling the hara; sitting in a secluded cell, it helps them make contact with the Unified Field. Try it sometime – on a bus, perhaps, or in a park. It will comfort you in *your* cell after you have made contact with the Uniformed Constabulary.

## Levitation

Savour this unique experience to the full. Tell your secretary you are not to be disturbed. Light up some incense, slip into a comfortable saffron shift, mount the filing cabinet and adopt the lotus position.

Close your eyes and quietly gibber your mantra to yourself. After a few moments you will feel youself rise gently and effort-lessly into the air, lifted aloft by two burly men in white jackets.

Smile beatifically at your terrified secretary as you glide off to the waiting ambulance.

## Dynamic Meditation

A truly cathartic experience which involves renting the air with screams for thirty minutes each morning. Invented by Tibetan monks to cope with the tensions of a monastic life in the High Himalayas. Sadly, they were eventually engulfed by an avalanche after a frenzied session during the spring thaw.

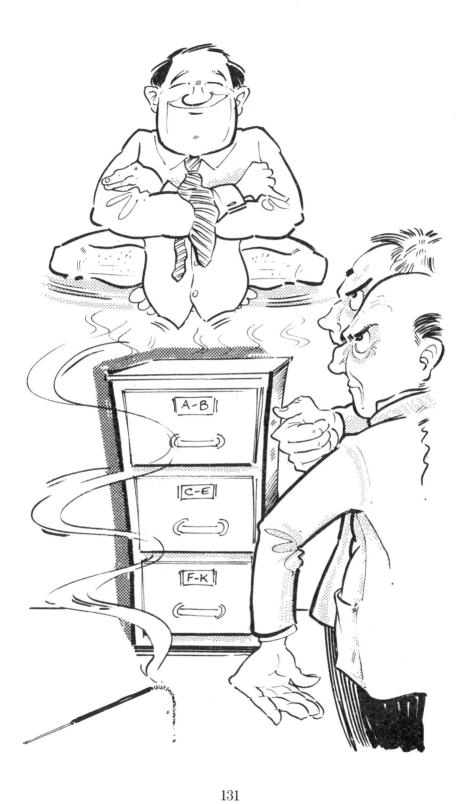

# Yoga

You may not know this, but each one of us possesses a coiled snake which lives in the base of our spine. Yoga exercises are designed to waken this serpent and lure it out into the open, presumably with a view to hitting it with a stick. Now if you're like me and have only just found out you've got this thing 'down there', you'll probably feel rather inclined to let sleeping dogs lie, so to speak.

However, apparently this is no mere grass snake but a reptile of cosmic proportions – presumably it's a bit like an anaconda, although it's difficult to see quite how it fits into your trousers. Anyway, by doing yoga exercises you sort of hypnotise it into life and it switches on all kinds of little light bulbs releasing energy you didn't know you had. Arthritis gets cured, blood gets beefed up and all without any drugs. Easy-peasy.

There are apparently 8½ million yoga positions originally described but some were safer than others so now there are only about 84. They can be divided into two categories – those *with* pogo sticks and those *without* pogo sticks.

Each exercise or 'Asana' is designed to help the body to accumulate vital energy or 'Prana' and to achieve serenity.

*Things you will need*
  *i* Prayer mat.
 *ii* Leotard and plimsolls.
*iii* Smelling salts.

*Easy ones*
**1** *Alternate Nostril Breathing.* Very simple and not at all strenuous. Much more dangerous on a pogo stick.
**2** *The Lion.* Crouch upright with your buttocks resting on your heels and your hands spread out on your thighs. Stick your tongue out as far as you can and stare wildly ahead. Done naked, this position is very good for frightening people coming up escalators.
**3** The *Plank of Wood*, the *Dead Vole* and the *Sleeping Bean Bag* are also undemanding exercises for the inexperienced aspiring yogi.

*Difficult Ones*
**1** *The Lotus.* Sitting cross-legged, wrap each heel firmly on to its opposite thigh. A pillow may help beginners. Bite on this when the pain gets unbearable.

**2** *The Praying Mantis.* Crouch on all fours with your buttocks high in the air. Inch your way on to the mantelpiece and wait for help to arrive.

**3** *The Mad Bat.* Placing the soles of your feet over your ears, gradually lift the weight on to your fingertips and raise yourself lightly into the air. Allow your buttocks to swing gently to and fro and pray that the vicar doesn't walk in unexpectedly.

# Acupuncture

An ancient and mysterious art invented by Chinamen around 3000 BC. Nobody knows what possessed them to stick pins in one another in the first place and the Chinese are very cagey about it, claiming they've forgotten. Since, as we all know, the Chinese have forgotten more than we've ever learnt, this is probably true. It may have happened by accident when they were busy forgetting how to invent knives and forks. How it works is a mystery, but no one now seriously doubts that correctly placed acupuncture needles can cure rheumatism, soothe runny eyes, ease pressure on sterling and bring about repeated orgasms and eclipses. Bodily tension ebbs away, warts drop off and lifelong addiction to Radio 1 ends overnight.

Ancient Taoist Chinamen discovered that we all contained some extremely inscrutable stuff called 'chi'. Not just *us* but *everything*. Nobody can see it, but it's there, slopping about the Universe causing everything to exist. (Before you snigger, just remember that these people invented telescopes while we were still bashing one another over the head with bits of rhino bone.) Just like the tide going in and out, this limpid invisible ectoplasm retreats and advances through the cosmos in a gentle rhythm familiar to us all as the 'the natural order of things'. In the body it flows along the International Dateline and ends at the speaking clock. Some meridians are 'Yang' meridians and others are 'Yin'. Others still are known as 'Yippee', 'Yoiks' and 'Tally Ho'.

Everything in the Universe is either Yin or Yang. Examples:

| *Yin* | *Yang* |
|---|---|
| Liver | Stomach |
| Heart | Bladder |
| Kidney | Large Intestine |

| *Yin* | *Yang* |
|---|---|
| Earth | Sun |
| Moon | Sky |
| Plain Yogurt | Credit Cards |
| BBC 2 | Pineapple Yogurt |
| Denture Adhesive | Radio 4 |
| Banana Republics | Capital Punishment |
| Liberty Bodices | Cobras |

By feeling your wrist, the acupuncturist can determine the imbalance of Yin and Yang in 436 languages. Carefully rubbing your skin with sweet and sour sauce, she will plunge a long sharp needle into a part of your anatomy remote from anywhere you know trouble to exist. This produces a response known to the Chinese as 'The Great Leap Forward'.

## The Naturopathic Approach

Among the many gifts Nature has bestowed upon our green planet, none is more welcome than the treasure trove she has given us for when we are sick. I refer, of course, to drugs. Consider the paradox of Mother Nature. For there she is – bounteous, caring, loving – giving us tablets to suck when our coronary arteries plug up with animal fat, pills to pop when normal surges of sex hormones threaten to lumber us with babies, and soothing capsules to calm frenzy whenever we feel like running amok on the Futures Market. Hard to believe that this same loving Mother Nature once set her noblest creature down in continents covered with impenetrable deciduous forests roaming with wild boar and flea-infested deer herds.

Sadly, Nature's blessings are not always appreciated. Even amongst my own patients there are those who seem to regard the drugs I dish out with scepticism bordering on suspicion. A careful explanation of side-effects often engenders a more positive response along the lines of, 'I'm not taking that muck.'

## Herbalism

In recent years, scurrilous stories about side-effects have caused many people to lose confidence in modern drugs. People have been turning in droves to the old-fashioned and natural ways of healing that were so successful in the times of Chaucer and the

Black Prince. Renewed interest in herbalism has seen the re-emergence of a long-lamented figure in medicine.

## The Old Crone

Although you can buy herbs from fancy health food shops, they are unlikely to be as efficacious and filthy as those obtained from an old crone. Genuine old crones live in dark stone hovels and have a framed certificate of agedness from the King.

Old crones don't like to be patronised. Go in, say 'Good morning, old crone,' and sit down on the earth. State your problem concisely in language she understands. For example:

'I am fuffering from ftale and obftinate grumes, fluxes of the belly and a touch of the Itch.'

She will then spit in your hand and demand money. Give her as much as she wants. She will take it and fall silent. This may be because she is thinking of a remedy or possibly she may have pegged it.

Write down her instructions carefully and piss off before you catch distemper or scrofula from the bits of old sacking hanging from the doorway. The remedy will be extremely old and should be followed to the letter, e.g.:

'Bruise fresh leaves of cuckoo pint gathered at dawn from the piggery. Grind in six garlic cloves, juice of ripened stinkwort and tincture of gambogie gum, using your pestle and mortar. Add droplets of pulverised skink and heat to Regulo 6. Set aside and whizz with fresh cow-dung in the food blender. Bake for three days.

(NB. Most courts consider this grounds for divorce on the basis of unreasonable behaviour and/or mental cruelty.)

The crucial last ingredient involves driving to a marsh in Buckinghamshire to scour the swamps for a rare species of Thyme dodder which grew there when the old crone was a girl . . . before they built Milton Keynes over it.

# Homeopathy

This fascinating doctrine was invented rather by accident by a crackpot German physician called Samuel Hahnemann, known to his learned colleagues as 'Screwball'.

Sadly Hahnemann was considered something of a joke in the academic circles of eighteenth-century Germany. . . . He did, how-ever, enjoy a huge reputation for his prowess with the pressure cooker, and for this reason his monthly scientific meetings, held in his University rooms, were guaranteed to be all-ticket affairs, with learned minds converging on Leipzig in the certain knowledge of a thumping good jam rolypoly.

These evenings were a great success. Blissfully impervious to the hoots of derision, the host would launch beamingly into his 'Seedcake Theory of Reproduction' whilst the cream of the German scientific community murdered fifteen vats of Brown Windsor soup and shovelled their way through his Daube de Boeuf.

Immune as he was to this insulting behaviour, even Hahnemann had his pride and eventually cracked. It happened one December evening when he was half-way through his paper on 'The Plasticine Liver'. Above the drone of indifference and the clatter of spoons on erudite dentures, the Emeritus Professor of Theology was heard to let slip an ill-chosen waspish remark about the sorbet.

Furious, Hahnemann stalked unnoticed from the dinner table, seized a bottle of arsenic, tossed it with onions, butter and parsley and threw it into the simmering Jambon Braise Morvandelle.

The results were remarkable. By the end of the evening the whole of the Humanities Faculty lay dead in their puddings, but the Professor of Theology seemed distinctly pukka and was duly arrested for the crime.

In the weeks before he perished on the scaffold, his rheumatism sped from his joints and, even more remarkably, his bladder ceased to empty itself emotionally during Evensong.

Hahnemann knew he had stumbled on something. For reasons he could not explain, the arsenic – diluted by piquant, aromatic sauce of mushrooms, braised in Pouilly Fuissé – had not killed the professor. It had made him better than he had ever been in his life.

Spurred on by this new theory, Hahnemann experimented with Filet de Poisson Poché laced with a trillionth part of strychnine. To his dismay, his invitations to supper were received with threadbare excuses from a suspicious academic community. . . .

'. . . Um . . . sorry, old bean . . . trying to lose some weight . . . er . . . allergic to garlic . . . must dash . . .'

In vain he pointed to his students, cured to a man of their revolting pustular acne.

He was shunned. Impoverished. Ostracised. The Napoleonic Wars came. . . . Asparagus ran short, lobster was unobtainable. Destitute, he was forced to continue his experiments with tap water. A billion parts of purified tap water to a grain of phosphorus, a pinch of mercury. Soon he ran out of poisons. Combing the woods for berries and funguses, his obsession for watering things down took a hold over him. His house was filled with vat after vat of remedies. He had remedies in the sink, in the bath and in the cistern. He even bled the radiators and filled them all with remedies.

Today, his encyclopaedic work – the *Materia Medica* – a glossary of poisons, metals, herbs and toenail clippings – is the Bible of the Modern Homeopath, though, regrettably, the 1,400-page appendix on Jellies and Trifles is missing from most translations.

## The Homeopathic Principle

This is the kind of strapping awarded to homeopaths when they've learnt the *Materia Medica* off by heart and undergone certain purification rituals.

Treating 'like with like' is the cornerstone of diagnosis and treatment. To find out what you are like, the homeopath may need to ask you all sorts of curious and improper questions about whether you sleep with your mouth open or your bum out of bed. In this they contrast with the polite concise manner of the orthodox doctor ('How are your bowels?' 'Fine.' 'Take these pills.').

The nature of the diagnosis differs too. The orthodox doctor will arrive at a crisp, descriptive diagnosis, e.g. 'blocked-up doings'. The homeopath, having interrogated you for two hours, will reach a more elaborate diagnosis of your personality type on which to base your remedy, e.g. Bland, innocuous, boring, colourless and stupid – treatment, grass cuttings; or Overbearing, greedy, smelly, oily and flatulent. Also stupid – treatment, nux vomica.

Homeopathy is especially good if you like people taking ages and ages arriving at the most accurate way to insult you.


## Music Therapy

As we have seen, using music to conjure torrents from stubborn bladders is just one example of the growing discipline of Music Therapy. So far, this ancient form of healing is enjoying its resurgence only at the fringes of medicine. One day, all this will change. Clinics for the waterworks will simply be incomplete unless they come kitted out with their own chamber orchestra. Fracture clinics will ring to the sound of the 'Anvil Chorus' being bashed out from the plaster room, and patients in the skin clinic will feel cheated unless they can scratch away to a bit of Vivaldi.

In time, surgical operations will only take place if there is an orchestra present. Private clinics will probably get in the Berlin Philharmonic, but the average punter may have to settle for the Salvation Army assisting at the removal of your gall bladder with a hearty rendition of 'Throw out the life-line', which will, nonetheless, be a comfort to your relatives, waiting anxiously in the foyer.

Hospital will become a happy place. No more angry scowls from grandpa when you dump him off at the Geriatric Day Centre – he'll be legging it down to join the Madrigal Therapy before you've had time to tuck in his shirt properly.

So what is so special about Music Therapy? Commonly, treatment is on the basis of treating 'like with like' – the rhythm and harmony of the piece mirroring the symptoms and enhancing the natural evolution and healing of the disorder.

Thus, for example, a *good-going boil* will mature naturally, to the swell of a symphony orchestra, enlarging steadily during the 'allegro' and usually beginning to throb and smoulder half-way into the 'andante non presso'. By the time the 'presto' is reached, it should be a nice rosy colour, slightly shiny, and shouldn't be pointed at anyone. The rest can be left to the final crash of the percussion section, leaving you to clean up the mess while someone changes the record.

*Never try self-treatment.* The 'Trumpet Voluntary', for example, can cause strangulation of previously trouble-free hernias. Always ask an expert. Here are some guidelines:

## Renal Colic
This excruciating condition needs something with good crescendoes and plenty of screaming. 'Madama Butterfly' is a good one, reserving the Mad Scene from 'Lucia di Lammermoor' for urgent cases.

## Constipation
Ravel's 'Bolero' is excellent, with 'Rule Britannia' a useful standby for patriotic sufferers. If desperate, Bach's 'Mass in B minor' is dynamite, as well as being most descriptive of the condition.

Whilst down at the other end, we ought to say a word about . . .

Overdoses are dangerous and vomiting should be induced with a gentle emetic, such as Dana, finishing the job by stomach pumping to some Debussy.

Finally, a word about Modern Music Therapy or 'Pop'. This is frowned upon by traditionalists, but I have to say that Marvin Gaye's 'I Heard it on the Grapevine' positively seduces wax out of the ears, while the lesser known 'I Caught it on the Clothesline' is certain to reduce priapism, which you can look up in a medical dictionary.

Work is still going on to establish the efficacy of 'I've Got You Under My Skin (scabies) 'I'm Going to Wash That Hare Right Out of My Man' (food poisoning) and 'You're Really a Part of Me' (tapeworm).

I've deliberately avoided sex, but I feel it must find a place, since Music Therapy has special virtues for all varieties of sexual difficulties.

Particularly recommended is 'Thus Spake Zarathustra', which is thoroughly uplifting in the treatment of impotence. If successful, this should be swiftly followed by a brisk polka and finally, after successful congress, you can both lie back and listen to the theme music from the 'Dam Busters'.

If you really can't face sex (again), say you've got a headache, call the doctor and quietly hum 'I Know that My Redeemer Liveth' while he's palpating your testicles.

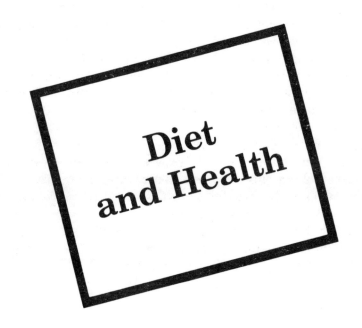

# Diet and Health

# Beginnings – Man as a 'Hunter-Gatherer'

As we all know, when *Homo sapiens* first descended from the trees, he was a 'hunter-gatherer'. What this means is that every morning the menfolk of the tribe went out from their caves at dawn, armed with spears and stone-axes, to hunt down mammoth elephants and woolly rhinoceros; and every evening the women-folk went out with large stone buckets and gathered up any remaining bits of the menfolk they could find.

The cave diet thus became a monotonous round of left-overs. Evenings were spent around the fire chewing over the day's casualties and fighting over the chief's wishbone. In time the men got uneasy about this pointless routine and, round about the second millennium, they downed tools and thereafter stayed in their caves daubing morose paintings.

Necessity being the Mother of Invention, the women turned their hands to cooking. First came the Rock Cake, a doughy concretion of flinty stones in mud, followed a little later by the Vol-au-vent, which was a total failure nutritionally but proved enormously popular for pelting warthogs.

## The Coming of the Seedpod

After millions of years of struggling with Nature, man realised that he was more than just a rough, uncouth savage. He was also a farmer. He learned how to till the land, plough it into furrows and scatter manure. For thousands of years he did this until somebody had the bright idea of putting some seeds in as well.

Before long, more imaginative farmers began to husband goats, pigs and chickens. All in all this led to a lot of ill-feeling with the womenfolk.

## The New Stone Age

Perhaps the most contented period of our history. Man, having survived the rigours of glaciers, volcanoes and pterodactyls, emerged as a skilled, cultured, gentle soul with a bone through his nose. Together with his wife and family, he dug drains, built houses, wove cloth and made earthenware pots. He became especially skilled with the bone, fashioning it into combs, fish-hooks and Royal Doulton teacups.

His diet was probably a model for healthy living:

Breakfast. Bilberry, nut and oatmix. Water.

143

Lunch. Wholemeal loaf, goat's cheese. Water.
Supper. Poached fish, cracked wheat and plums. Water.
Nightcap. Assorted berries. Water.

In contrast, today's noble savage might expect:

Breakfast. Coffee, six sugars. Cigarette. Bacon butty in the car on the way to the shareholders' meeting.
Midmorning. Mars Bar.
Lunch. Beer. Pâté bap. Crisps/pork scratchings.
Tea. Cakey and a mug of tepid, brown sugary water.
Supper. Steak and kidney pud, chips, ketchup. Treacle tart and cream. ½ bottle of Côte de Beaune-Villages.
Midnight. Raid fridge for Auntie Maud's home-made chocolate boggis cake.
2 a.m. Rennies.

Man has adapted to the privations of a twentieth-century diet by becoming quite extraordinarily fat.

## How Fat is Too Fat?

| | *Slightly Overweight* | *Distinctly Pudgy* | *Moutainous* |
|---|---|---|---|
| You are able to slip with minimum difficulty into | a large pair of trousers | an ample kaftan | a double garage |
| In bed you are | cuddly | all right provided you don't roll over | unable to roll over without calling the AA. |
| Measuring your waist requires | a long tape measure | a clothesline | a quantity surveyor |
| In bed you sleep under | a very big sheet | a king-size duvet | a tarpaulin |
| Your favourite nibbles are | cashew nuts | suet pudding | Herefords |

# How to Lose Weight

Most experts nowadays recommend diets high in natural fibre and roughage. Fibre rushes through the intestine a bit like stampeding bicyclists on the Tour de France; you'll notice a lot of rushing wind and you'll probably need bicycle clips.

Many special high fibre diets now exist:

*The G-Plan Diet.* A good Habitat sofa, pulpued and shredded, contains all the fibre you need without an ounce of absorbable nourishment. Less monotonous if varied with colourful Heal's cushion covers or a Laura Ashley duvet.

*The Crispbread/Branbud Experience.* What this lacks in variety for the tastebuds it makes up for in decibels. A very noisy, crunchy diet. Armed with a good set of molars you can mimic the reoccupation of the Rhineland over breakfast. Digestion is also a noisy affair, reminiscent of heaving sluice gates, very heavy plugs being pulled, and gurgling tidal locks opening and shutting prior to the passage of a large tug round about 11 o'clock.

*The Wholefood Purgative Meringue.* Made from unpolished rice, crunchy sunflower seeds, ground-up eggshell and slithers of bamboo. Guaranteed to make your mouth really water and very probably bleed.

*Microdiets.* A drastic measure devised in Cambridge to cope with intractably bunged-up dons. Many of these liquid diets are expensive but the nutritional content is scientifically balanced from years of experimenting with sheep dips.

## Cleansing and Purifying Diets

A lot depends on how cleansed you want to be. For a really good spring-clean round the U-bend and complete respray of your liver and entrails, you will first have to give up fried food, meat, coffee, tea, sugar, alcohol, eggs, salt and dairy products. It's a bit like being weaned off a life-support machine. The first five minutes are usually the worst.

*The Grape Fast.* This is just to let your liver know you mean business. It is quite surprising how monotonous grapes can seem after three days. Practise peeling them in your mouth and draping the skins over your teeth so they all look green and black.

145

Probably you will have mastered this by mid-morning. Try sticking the pips together and see if you can make a facsimile of Nelson's flagship. Then pretend you are Moby Dick and chomp ravenously through the keel with all hands on deck.

*Brown Rice.* A week or ten days of this will have you screaming for the grapes to be brought back.

*Raw Vegetables, Brewer's Yeast and Garlic.* After a fortnight's privation, your system will have earned this bold splash of colour. Make the most of it. Enjoy that wicked bit of swede to the full. Feel that watercress scorching the crud off the stomach lining. Delicious! Crack open the prune juice and live dangerously.

By the end of this regime your splanchnic mesocolon will be sparkling like the Crystal Palace. Your plasma will waft melodiously around long-forgotten channels and sumps, and glistening lymph will bathe your viscera in vitamins, garlic and herbal tea. The mere sight of a pork chop will revolt you. You may well want to celebrate with some coitus.

*Aphrodisiacs.* Reeking of garlic as you do, you will probably need some assistance from Nature's pleasure palace. The following concoction can be ground over the oyster bisque already chilling in one of your sweetheart's slippers.
1 Ginseng.
2 Vitamin E.
3 Powdered rhino horn.
4 Old man's beard.
5 Jasmine blossom and betel juice.
6 Old man's rhino.

# Food Allergy

A modern affliction causing rashes, arthritis, dyslexia, hyperactive children and most cases of homicide and shoplifting. Common culprits are red meat, caffeine, food additives, eggs, Navarin of lamb and Clafouti aux pommes.

Many previously inexplicable phenomena are now known to be due to food allergy. Allergy to strawberries was probably responsible for the Second Punic War and an injudicious Kentucky Fried Chicken almost certainly caused Yamamato's beastly migraine just before he unleashed bombs on Pearl Harbour.

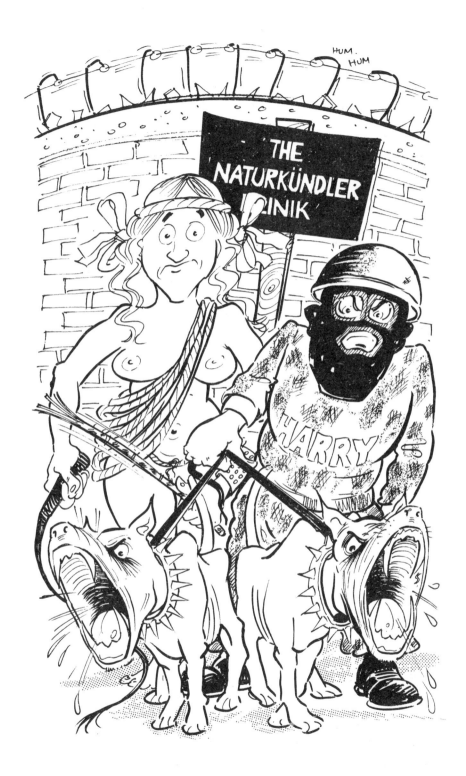

Infants are especially susceptible to old-fashioned bosoms that dole out breast milk – babies never used to behave like that. Toddlers and school children are notoriously allergic to chocolate, artificially coloured juices and bright sweeties. Many go berserk an hour or two later – usually coinciding with normal meal times; hurling potato and greens round the walls, spitting and gagging are typical symptoms of food allergy.

## E Numbers

E Numbers are code names for food additives, colourings, preservatives, etc. They are believed by some to be the twentieth-century equivalent of the black rat as a menace to health. Others think this is an exaggeration. Many naturopathic food freaks would probably prefer the black rat to tartrazine (E102) as it goes quite well with custard and doesn't excite the children so much. Junk foods contain lots and lots of E numbers, which is why they look so pretty and appetising. Personally, I think we should have more E numbers and fewer naturopathic fruit-cakes.

Here are some I can really recommend if you fancy stopping up all night hoovering and singing:

E106 – ethyl ester of beta-apro-8-caortenoic acid. (E 106 is much more convenient as you can get lots and lots of it in a tin of plums and still manage to fasten the lid down.)
E155 – a chocolate brown extravaganza excellent for cultivating enormous confluent zits.
E142 – 'Brilliant Lissamine Green'. Capable of sending you really potty. Nero is said to have eaten his way through a barrowload of bright green jelly just before he burnt down Rome.
E410 – Locust bean gum. Used for thickening food and mending lorries. Somewhat constipating.

## Health Farms

Health Farms are places you go to get right away from the stress and strain of your unhealthy workaday existence. Far from the madding crowd, the junk-food and the pollution, you can pamper yourself back to fitness and health.

The Naturkündler Klinik in Hampshire, run by ex-Congo veteran Captain 'Mad Harry' Doberman-Pitt and his charming wife Hildegarde, offers unique macrobionic weekends in acres of unspoilt parkland, protected from the public gaze by an electric fence.

The day begins early – usually 4 a.m. – with a nude run through mixed deciduous woodland, pursued by the dogs. This is followed by two hours of PE on the lawns to rousing martial music supervised by Hildegarde, who is even more striking naked than when she's in her rope get-up.

Breakfast in the Refectory is a cheerful interlude when you can get to know your chums – over a cup of lemon juice and a bucket of the Klinik's famous muesli, made from wheat germ, hulled sunflower seeds, sultanas and beetroot.

The Pump Room is a big attraction. The mineral water – rich in manganese and calcium – is believed to come from an underground spring, thence through very old zinc pipes before it finally arrives at the water cannon. The hose-down that follows is truly exhilarating. Freezing cold jets of aqua vitae hurl you screaming around the marble floors for nearly an hour, tossing you against the ceilings till the water level eventually rises enough to enable you to shriek for help through the metal grid.

The Solarium is in the hottest part of the garden. It's a simple design of corrugated metal very similar to the one used in 'Bridge over the River Kwai' to bake Colonel Bogey. Temperatures reach an invigorating 105°F, enabling you to sweat out poisonous wastes in complete privacy.

By the time they drag you out, your body will be rid of muscle tension, totally limp and flaccid, but still breathing feebly. Toning up the muscles follows immediately, beginning with a soap-and-water enema and followed by a brisk massage by Dobson; Dobson probably isn't his real name as he's a twenty stone wrestler from Kowloon. He's got very gentle hands for a man of his size – very soft and sensitive with exquisitely manicured fingers. Dobson prefers to use his very large horny feet to massage you, stamping up and down your spine and then sitting on your head.

Lunch. By now you are ravenous. Just as well the Captain has prepared enough Garbanzo Bean Pilaf to feed the Red Army. If you've still got an empty corner somewhere, his Carrageen Moss Pudding and carrot juice will give you bags of energy for an afternoon of rounders and a whip round the assault course.

The Assault Course. You are allowed to do this in your vest and pants, mainly to give you the edge over the piranha fish. Special features include – The Wall, The Hill, The Big Jump, the Bottomless Chasm and the Mangling Cupboard.

Evening. After an hour's meditation in a darkened box, Dobson returns to give you a quick rub-down with sandalwood and rancid

Tibetan butter, prior to a wrestling match and the insertion of some herbal suppositories.

Supper of carob brownies and pumpkin seeds induces a healthy fit of vomiting, emptying the intestine of all remaining toxins.

After Lights Out at 9 p.m. Hildegarde goes from room to room giving individual bend and stretch exercises or a choice of thrashings.

## Cost
About £600 all in. No pets, transistor radio or ethnic minorities please.

## Some Views On The Creation

As a busy general practitioner, one doesn't really have time for religion, but in more reflective moments, I do wonder whether the body, with all its miraculous intricacies, was put together as a result of millions of years of natural selection, or by God, who, as even non-believers would concede, must have been awfully bright and would have simply sailed through medical school.

So who was the Great Architect? Who holds the patent? I've been giving this a lot of thought recently and perhaps I can best illustrate them for you in the following tabulated form.

| FOR GOD | FOR DARWIN |
|---|---|
| **1.** The complexities and marvels of the brain, heart, kidneys and liver. Is it conceivable that these wonders could have been contrived by mutation and chance? | On the other hand, we have feet, armpits, ear-wax and naval-fluff. Are we to believe that God sat down and invented these things? And for Heaven's sake, what for? |
| **2.** The mind. Surely, this undiscovered and undiscoverable labyrinth, secret and inviolable, could not merely have evolved. What about Mozart, Einstein, Leonardo and Shakespeare? | What about Gary Glitter and The Troggs? |

150

**3.** Man is but one of thousands of species that has to take his place in a world of unsurpassed beauty and variety.

Humming birds of shimmering green, hovering above explosions of orange bougainvillea and yellow jacaranda; the feline grace of the predatory leopard, stalking the lisson and innocent gazelle . . .

All that may sound very poncy and nice, but it has to be said that a great obstacle lies in the path of the Divine Creationalists in the shape of the giant slug.

Are we seriously to consider that His Nibbs spent a great deal of, let's face it, what was only six days, coming up with something that spends it's life squidging around under cabbage-leaves, contributing to life's rich pattern by leving a long streak of gunge trailing behind it?

**3.a.** On the subject of the opposite, did it ever occur to the Darwinists that God *did* invent slugs, but they simply just didn't come out right?

And for God's sake, no-one's perfect.

**4.** So who wrote the Bible then??

Ermm . . .

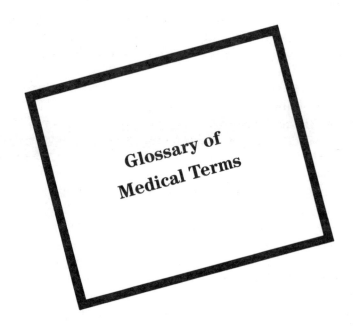

Glossary of
Medical Terms

*Dentist.* Someone who behaves like a doctor, but drives a Porsche.

*Errors of Judgement.* An occasional occurrence e.g. taking out the wrong kidney. Hospitals are generally very good about this sort of thing and get you back as soon as possible to take out the other one.

*Fertility Drugs.* Very important break-through. Includes 'Baby Bio' and Rooting Powder.

*Funeral.* Do not ask doctor to come to your funeral. It's like asking your defending council to visit you in jail.

*House-call.* An outlandish demand on doctor's time. It had better be serious.

*Hydrotherapy.* Treatment designed to quell hysteria by throwing you in water.

*Medical Emergency.* A distressing time for doctor when he thinks he's going to get sued.

*Miracle Cure.* Has a proven record with rats and monkeys.

*Pain Threshold.* The point at which other people think you ought to start hurting.

*Physiotherapy.* Treatment designed to bring life back to tired bodies. A week down the quarry generally works a treat.

*Prolapse.* An introductory passage to a medical book.

*Receptionist.* The medical equivalent of the Berlin Wall. Every surgery should have a Berlin Wall.

*Revolutionary New Drug.* Has a proven record with rats and monkeys.

*Rigor Mortis.* Consult your doctor immediately. It's likely to get worse.

*Rising Damp.* A distressing condition of late middle-age. Particularly unpleasant when it meets Descending Dank on its way down.

*Rubber Gloves.* Worn when having to poke about in dark places. Also for washing up.

*Skeleton Service.* Doctor's not *always* on call.

*Suppository.* A collective noun for medical instruments e.g. A suppository of tongue depressers.

*Test Tube Baby.* Babies that are 'grown on' in a test-tube. Tend to grow up fairly thin and somewhat claustrophobic.

*TNT.* Tri-nitro toluene. Should not be confused with PMT.

*Thermometer.* A useful device. Often stuck in the mouth. Stops the patient yapping while doctor tries to think what's wrong with you.

*Traditional Remedy.* Tried and tested and hasn't worked for hundreds of years.

*'Waterworks'.* A term often used by doctor to denote the goings on below the Plimsoll Line. He might even mention your 'plumbing', for the same reason.

# Bibliography and suggested reading

| | |
|---|---|
| **Doctor Zhivago** | B. Pasternak |
| **Randy Doctors on the Job** | Various |
| **A Life in Medicine** | C. Crippen |
| **The Bacillus Joke Book** | L. Pasteur |
| **Freemasonry and Fungi** | M. Lodge |
| **Purges and Splurges** | Burgess and Sturges |
| **Unravelling the Crick** | Helix and Watson |
| **East of Sewage** | Min. Public Works |
| **Ice Cold in Ajax** | Admiral Sir Humphrey Tewfick (Deceased) |
| | |
| **Communicable Diseases** | Anon |
| **The Tapeworm Year Book** | Thames Valley Worm Society |
| **Fibroids Can be Fun** | C. Sweet (Unpublished) |
| **Renal Colic and the Punic Wars** | 1954 Boy's Own Annual |
| **Adventures with Skin Tags** | Lord de Moyne (Banned) |
| **Anthrax for All the Family** | Friends of the Earth Annual |
| **Acne for Beginners** | C. Sweet (Unpublished) |

# PS

I feel very humble that through the aegis of this modest little book, I have been able to share with you the magic and majesty that is the human body. Well some of them anyway. I need only add that if any of you are passing by my neck of the woods, please do not hesitate to pop in for a cup of tea and a private consultation. You can be rest assured that without all those horrid NHS-type patients gumming up the works, you are guaranteed my absolute and devoted attention at the rate of 22 guineas per hour. And as a special introductory offer, if you have *two* diseases, you will get the first one treated absolutely free of charge!

As you know, my terms of employment prevent me from advertising, but my wife is quite happy to take calls on Hillview 8246. Be sure to mention that you're paying through the private nose scheme.

If you have time and happen to have a pen in your hand, why don't you just fill in the little application form which you'll find below . . . That's right . . . see below. Now, cut it out with your little scissors and send it off as soon as you can – registered post will be fine.

Thank you so much. You know, I feel as if I've been speaking to you in very much a personal way and I trust that this book has, in some funny way, brought us all a little closer. Because, you know, medicine has taught me a lot of things, but I think its main one has been that although our bodies differ, from the beautiful to the frankly revolting, we are still brothers and sisters and absolutely equal in the eyes of our Maker.

That's *HILLVIEW 8246*.

I ............................................................ wish to become a private patient.

My annual income is ........................................................................................

My house is worth around £...............................................................................

I voted ............................................................ in the last general election

I think doctors are ...........................................................................................